In The
CARE of
STRANGERS

Linda Pischke
Dr. Calvin Langmade

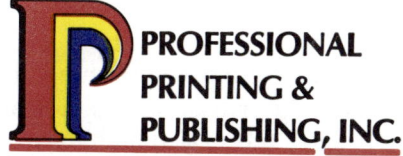

PROFESSIONAL PRINTING & PUBLISHING, INC.

P.O. Box 5758 · Bossier City, LA 71171-5758
318-746-6880 · 1-800-551-8783 · FAX 318-746-6995
Web Site: http://www.ppandp.com
E-mail: order@ppandp.com

ISBN 0-929442-37-7

Professional Printing & Publishing, Inc.
P.O. Box 5758
Bossier City, LA 71171-5758
318/746-6880
WATS 1-800/551-8783 - FAX 318/746-6995
Web Site: http://www.ppandp.com
E-mail: order@ppandp.com

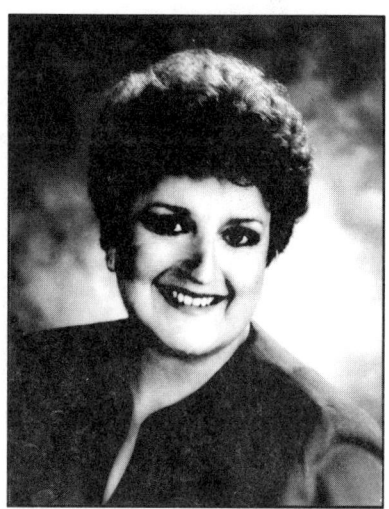

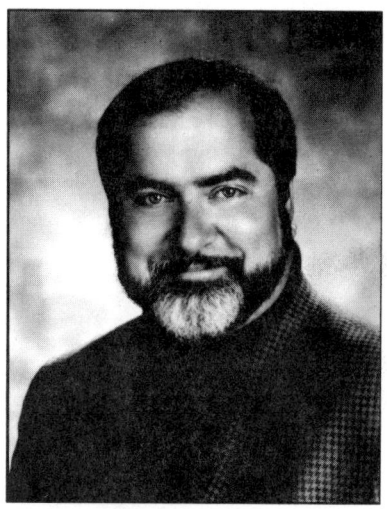

Linda Pischke is a licensed social worker and the Director of Resident Services at a senior facility in Waukesha, Wisconsin. She counsels families in matters related to placement and implements life enrichment programs for residents. Linda has been a guest lecturer on subjects related to residents' rights, crafts for special needs, and resident community groups. Her first published book, *Keeping In Touch With The Community, A Guide To Resident Volunteer Programs*, is available through Professional Printing & Publishing, Inc.

Dr. Calvin Langmade is a clinical psychologist in private practice in Milwaukee, Wisconsin. He received his doctorate in Clinical Psychology form Rosemead School of Psychology in Los Angeles, California. Dr. Langmade has consulted with families and residents in the long-term care setting. He is an adjunct graduate faculty member of the psychology department of Wheaton College and is a frequent speaker to business and community groups on issues that impact individuals in daily living.

Both authors can be contacted through Dr. Langmade's self-help Web site, Doc In The Box (http//www.docinthebox.com)

Acknowledgments

The contributions of many people have made this book possible. We would like to express our gratitude to the following individuals for their generous gifts of time and knowledge: nursing home residents who told us their stories, family members who shared the difficulties of dealing with aging parents, Reverend Richard Engen for his insight into parent/child role reversal, those who participated in focus groups and individual interviews, and our co-workers whose expert knowledge of eldercare helped us bring it all together. Thanks to Kathy Kaufman, our mentor and friend, who kept telling us, "You can do it"; JoAnne Konkel for proofreading and helping us prepare the manuscript; and our families and friends who supported us, cheered us on, and listened patiently to our endless discussion of this work. Special thanks to Dr. Victor Oliver for his encouragement in the early days of this manuscript.

A special thanks to
Bethany L. Kopp
Muralist & Designer
for her talent and creativity
as so beautifully displayed
on the cover of our book.

Preface

This book is about life on the inside. It is a rare and intimate glimpse of a world that most of us fear, few of us discuss and some of us have never seen. It is about a community of individuals who, for a time, are separated from society while they take on the task of growing old and facing death in a nursing home. This is a story about love and commitment, a story of families and the strangers who serve them.

In September of 1994, we met for the first time to discuss the possibility of writing a book about nursing homes. At that time, we were privileged to work in one of the finest long-term care facilities in the United States. Our original purpose for this manuscript was to assist families in the process of selecting a good facility. We felt that everyone should have expert guidance in negotiating the best possible care for his or her loved ones.

Many of the families who came to us for advice already knew how to choose a good nursing home for their parents. What they sought from us was comfort and reassurance. When we asked ourselves, "What makes this process so difficult?" we had the basis for an entirely different kind of book. The question was not only about whether families selected a good nursing home or a bad one. It was about how they dealt with the grief and guilt of placing loved ones in the care of strangers.

In our search for answers, we discovered that the nursing home community is comprised of a remarkable group of human beings, each with a lifetime of stories to tell. The stories in this book are true. We have changed names and identifying details to protect the privacy of those involved. One story, however, has not been changed. At the request of Patsy, we have left everything just as she told it to us. In her words, "I have no regrets. I have nothing to hide."

We began our research with focus groups. These consisted of individuals in the community, who volunteered to share their beliefs about issues related to aging. The first group, Generation X, involved participants eighteen to twenty one. The second group included individuals thirty to fifty-years old. The third was made up of persons sixty and over who were served by a community meal program. All group members were asked a similar set of questions. They discussed their perceptions of growing old, what they felt it would be like to live in a nursing home, and the losses related to the aging process. A final focus group consisted of family members belonging to a local chapter of Citizens' Advocates for Nursing home Reform. In this group, we examined the problems families face with placement and the negative aspects of long-term care.

After meeting with the focus groups, we conducted one-on-one interviews with residents currently living in nursing homes, their family members and their caregivers. Additional contributions for this work came from nurses, administrators and social workers.

The long-term care setting is home to many individuals. Persons with various forms of debilitating illnesses are often cared for in this environment. While our study concerns the needs of the elderly, the principles in this book apply to any residents who live in institutions.

Our desire to write this book developed while working together in a long-term care facility. We were the "strangers" to whom families entrusted their loved ones. In helping them deal with their grief and guilt, we came to realize that death and human frailty are subjects of great discomfort to all of us. In the process, we also learned that the comfort we seek is to be found in God's word. We invite you to be open-minded as we explore this unique community.

Introduction

The American family has undergone dramatic changes since World War II and the emergence of the Baby Boomer generation. The "needs" of this generation have made a tremendous impact on the economy and our society as a whole. It is the largest and wealthiest generation in American history with more professional business people, higher wages, larger houses and more toys, along with a growing population of unemployed and homeless. As a result, the physical makeup of the family unit and our beliefs about what constitutes family life have changed by their very definition.

The focus of this generation is on self-fulfillment and financial gain, sometimes at the expense of others. Concern about what benefits the family as a whole, has been replaced by a "what's-in-it-for-me?" philosophy. In fact, it was during the 1980s that Baby Boomers were labeled the "Me Generation" and adopted as their motto, "The one who dies with the most toys wins!" Our society's values have been so altered by these "needs" that we marry at a later age, choose to have fewer children, and welcome divorce as a solution to our family problems. Single-parent families have become as common as the traditional Judeo-Christian family model, that has been the foundation of our society for hundreds of years.

The Baby Boomer lifestyle, often dependent on two incomes, makes it difficult for us to support larger families or to meet the physical, financial and emotional needs of children and the elderly. Once valued family members, they have become an inconvenience and a financial burden. It is a growing trend to place our young children in day-care centers to be raised by individuals who have no kinship to them.

Likewise, as our human life span increases, we seek more solutions to eldercare, such as day care, assisted living, and long-term care facilities. Thus, we separate our very young and very old from the family unit and place them in the care of strangers.

This shift from the importance of the family, as a unit, to a focus on personal financial security and well being has taken its toll. The economic and emotional stresses that exist in the late twentieth century are beginning to undermine the very foundation of our society. For years, we have listened to talk-show hosts and pop psychologists discuss what is and what is not healthy about our family life. The never-ending parade of the bizarre and unusual on such shows has resulted in a loss of value for the traditional and, ultimately, a loss of being rooted in the family.

Despite our concern with family problems, we rarely discuss or acknowledge the personal needs of the aging. We comfort ourselves by talking about Social Security and other financial programs. We demand that nursing homes are designed to accommodate our idea of affluence, and we enact cumbersome nursing-home reform to still our consciences. But few of us become personally involved in the day-to-day issues of care, because we fear the inevitable, our own aging and death.

In the mid-1990s, Baby Boomers began to enter what is called "fifty-plus," the late middle-adult years. With each passing year, the numbers in this group will grow rapidly, and they will face critical financial and personal issues which will have long-term consequences affecting their retirement years. Baby Boomers will begin to deal with the needs of their aging parents and their own fears about growing old and dying. The demands for eldercare will be greater than ever before and will continue to increase as this generation ages. The children of Baby Boomers, in their significantly fewer numbers, will not be able to bear the financial or physical burden.

It was for this reason that we chose to write a book about long-term care and the families, caregivers and residents who make up this community of individuals. It is not our intent to be judgmental of the choices that families make or to offer solutions. It is merely a place to begin in our awareness of this misplaced, and often forgotten, part of our society.

Table of Contents

  Marge's Rehab Journal • A glimpse of nursing home
  life as seen through the eyes of a younger woman
  who is there for short-term rehabilitation

  Arthur • The Crisis Of Aging • The Last Thing We
  Talk About • Coming To Terms With Growing Old

  Mama • The Sandwich Generation • Family
  Traditions And Eldercare • The Stigma Of Nursing
  Homes • The Nursing-Home Decision

  Jake • Our Responsibility To Family • The Good
  Old Days • No Easy Answers • Facing The Facts

This book is dedicated to
our parents

Andrew and Gladys Young
Oliver and Mary K. Langmade

CHAPTER ONE

Golden Days -
A Journal

You should defend those
who cannot help themselves.
Yes, speak up for the
poor and helpless,
and see that they get justice.

(Proverbs 31:8)
The Living Bible

Marge's Rehab Journal

January 17- Claire called from Arizona last night. I told her that my foot wasn't healing as fast as expected and that Dr. Harris wants me to go to a rehab center for about two weeks. She and John offered to cut their trip short and take care of me at home, but I said, "Nonsense. The insurance pays for this, and I'll be home before you are." She said, "Keep a journal, Mom. You always liked to write, and it will make the days go faster."

January 19- Admission day, 10:00 a.m. My insurance company gave me two choices. One had an opening - Golden Days Health Care and Rehabilitation Center (alias nursing home). Dear God, I don't belong here. This is supposed to be a place for old people. I'm sixty-two. I've got all my senses. I drive a car. I work. As a matter of fact, I'm very good at what I do. I'm so different from all the others. A social worker read me my rights. They also do that when you go to jail.

1:00 p.m.- Hundreds of questions, a body check, papers to sign. "You'll be eating in the main dining room. This is where you sit. It's part of your rehab." What was it that the Resident's Rights list said about choices? My tablemates all had bibs. I was offered one and accepted. It's hard to eat in a wheelchair with your foot elevated in front of you. I dribbled Sloppy Joe mix on myself and smiled at the woman across from me. She was being fed Sloppy Joe puree. Her name is Martha, and she looks to be about ninety.

8:00 p.m.- Spent the afternoon in physical therapy. They told me it was wonderful to have someone they could really talk to. It's a warm, kind place. There was a soft hum of voices and laughter as we were put through our exercises. One little grandma whimpered like a puppy when they gently moved her arms and legs. Another slapped and tried to bite. I was happy to learn that a third of the residents here go back home. It turns out that ninety-year-old Martha is my roommate. She was in bed and asleep by 7:30. Poor thing, she looked so tired. I asked my nurse aide, Genie, to pull the privacy curtain so I could have my light on to read. Tomorrow, I'll have a phone. My dear neighbor, Jan, is bringing me more clothes and a small TV.

January 21- They get me up at 6:30. It's part of my rehab. This morning I got a shower and shampoo on an open bottom, tubular plastic chair with wheels. It looked like that cheap lawn furniture they sell at the state fair, the stuff that's made out of PVC pipe. My aide was Cindy, a very sweet young girl who offered me the privacy of washing myself, but forgot to close the bathroom door.

January 23- A wheelchair gives you a very different view of the world. In the hospital, it was just a means of getting from my bed to another location, like X-ray or therapy. Here, I live in it, at least until I can bear weight on my foot. Some of the staff sits or bends to meet my eyes when we talk. Some just look down on me. From my chair, I gaze into faces. They don't always know that I'm here, even when I speak.

January 24- 12:00 a.m.- It's so hot in here. Sometimes I have trouble sleeping. Caroline walks up and down the halls looking for her mother. Martha's breath rattles in the night. She's checked and changed every two hours. The night nurse helped herself to a piece of Martha's chocolate. I wonder what else she has taken. "Dear Lord, bless Martha and all the other people here. Amen.... And God, touch the heart of that nurse who thinks our things belong to her." Pastor Gunderson visited today. He said this is a good nursing home, if you have to be in one. Several of our church members have lived...and died here.

January 25- Sunday. I went to Mass on Thursday. Today, we had bingo. I guess most churches are too busy to do a Sunday service. Maybe they think it doesn't matter because some of us are confused anyway. Martha's daughter came after lunch today. Martha had food spills on her dress and crumbs in her lap, and she asked, "Who are you?" three times. After ten minutes, her daughter gave her a kiss on the cheek and said, "See you next week, Mom." Then she turned to me. "I guess it's for the best. She doesn't remember about the cancer." I wanted to mention the chocolate, but changed my mind.

January 26- I asked for an extra piece of fruit at breakfast. The kitchen girl very nicely told me it wasn't on my diet card. I asked to see the dietitian. "She'll be in on Tuesday, dear," was her reply. I said, "I've been a diabetic for 20 years. I ought to know if I can have an extra piece of fruit or not!" If I had a dollar for every time someone called me Honey or Dear, I could take a trip when I get out of here. I want to scream, "My name is Marge, please use it!"

January 27- Ten years ago, my mother lived in a nursing home. When we went to visit, she didn't know us any more. I wish now that I had taken the time to sit at her side and hold her hand the way John W. sits with his father. He comes every day to feed him lunch and bring a special treat for dessert. His dad never says a word, but John is there.

January 28- I had to wait 45 minutes for a bedpan this morning. My aide, Christine, said they were working short. I scolded her for taking so long. I'm crabby and sick of waiting for everything. This is such a waste of time. We lose so much here. Not just our homes and our possessions, but privacy and choices and dignity. I get to leave next week. What about the others? What do they get?

January 29- Which world do I belong to, Lord? Last month I was part of the outside. I lived alone. I took myself to the bathroom and ate when I wanted to. Today, I'm a resident and all the things I took for granted are coveted. Are we really so separate? A change of circumstance and we're on the other side.

February 1- 5:30 a.m.- Martha and I will both be leaving today. When they checked her at 4:00 a.m., the rattles had stopped. It's so quiet now. The nurse insisted that I get up and sit in the dining room until the undertaker comes. I'm not afraid to be with her body. She's in the arms of Jesus, smiling and young again. My mother died alone.

CHAPTER TWO

Seasons

*To everything
there is a season
and a time
for every purpose
under heaven.
A time to be born
and a time to die.*

(Ecclesiastes 3:1-2)
King James

Arthur

The smell of urine hit me as I pushed my way through the double doors of Three Southwest at the VA hospital. It was the first day of my geriatric rotation, and I was late for a group. I wiped the sweat from my forehead with the back of my hand, resisting the urge to cover my nose.

The other interns had warned me, "Hope ya got a strong stomach when you work geropsyche, Cal. The smell of that place is gonna stop you right in your tracks. And just wait 'till you play the parachute game. You'll get a real laugh out of that one."

The smell grew stronger. As I headed down the narrow hallway with its gray walls and black-and-white checkered floor, I was reminded of a morning ten years earlier, at the Boone County Poor Home. Our youth group was required to do the Sunday service and hymn sing. It was my first view of institutional living. The sight of old people sitting in wheelchairs with nothing to do shocked me. The place had the disgusting smell of dirty diapers and, with some embarrassment, I remember promising that I would kill myself before I'd ever live in an old folks' home.

At the desk I maneuvered around a tangle of wheelchairs. It didn't appear as if things had changed much in nursing homes since I was a kid. One elderly veteran, apparently unable to right himself, was leaning so far over the left arm of his chair that his hand almost touched the floor. A puddle of urine had formed beneath him.

Another grabbed at me, "Mister, can ya get me outa here? I gotta catch the bus and go to work."

His plea was interrupted by a younger voice.

"Dr. Langmade? We've been waiting for you." A nervous young man walked up to me, placed his hands on his hips, and glared. "You have delayed our afternoon exercise. I'm Bill, the occupational therapist. I lead this group. Please join us."

We entered a large sitting room directly across from the nurses' station, where eight or nine elderly men sat in wheelchairs. The chairs had been placed around a brightly colored circle of fabric that lay stretched out on the floor. In the center of the fabric was a small beach ball.

Bill walked around the outside of the group, picking up the edge of the fabric as he went and placing it in the hands of each group member. I was directed to pull up a chair and take my place between two of the men.

"This must be the infamous parachute game," I thought.

Introductions were ignored. A television blasted behind me to my right; World Series, Dodgers vs. Yankees. Frankly, the ball game seemed more appropriate to me.

"Okay, peeepul," Bill shouted, flapping his arms up and down. "Let's exercise those muscles! I absolutely must have your cooperation. EVERYONE lift up as high as you can. Make that ball bounce up and down. That's it! Very gooood!"

I felt stupid playing this child's game. The gentleman to my left mumbled something under his breath, let go of the parachute, and stretched back in his wheelchair to get a better view of the game. The chair, too small for his tall frame, almost tipped over.

"Arthur, let's pay attention here," Bill scolded him. "We must all work together."

Arthur muttered, "Stupid idiot."

One of the Vets echoed, "Work together, work together."

"Aw, shut up Harry. Do you have to repeat everything?" said another.

"Puleeze, let's not fight, gentlemen. We're here to exercise." The impatience in Bill's voice created even more disruption and unwanted comments.

"All right, if you don't appreciate my time and energy, we'll quit for today." Bill walked up to me. "It's impossible to do this thankless job with so little help."

Bill dismissed the group and went to do his charting at the nurses' station. Those who were able moved on to other things. A half-dozen men remained parked in their wheelchairs, unattended. I decided to stay.

I walked over to Arthur who had positioned himself in front of the television set. He was talking and gesturing to an unseen person on his right. Occasionally, he would stop and move his mouth as if he was chewing. He needed a shave and a bath. I pulled up my chair and asked if I could watch the game with him. He shrugged his shoulders and moved his wheelchair closer to me.

"Like baseball, do you?" I asked, not sure how to start a conversation with a demented person.

"Yup." Arthur leaned forward and spit on the floor in front of us.

"I've played a little, as a kid," I urged, hoping to keep the conversation going.

"Me, too," Arthur said, continuing to stare at the TV.

"When was that?"

"Long time ago." He chewed and spit again.

"What do you think of Los Angeles?" I asked.

"Don't care much for these players."

"What don't you like about them?"

Arthur didn't respond. I wondered if he'd heard me and tried another question. "Tell me what baseball was like when you were a young man."

"It ain't like it used to be."

"Why not?" I asked.

For the first time Arthur turned to look at me. "Cuz I ain't play'n."

"You played professional baseball?"

"Yup." He looked back at the TV.

"Where did you play?"

"Majors." He spit a little further this time.

I paused, wondering if I should pursue this conversation. Was I encouraging the delusions of a confused man? Would this serve any purpose or would it upset him? Curious, I took a chance.

"What was the most memorable moment in your career?"

Arthur turned to me again, studying my face as if to decide whether I could be trusted. He stopped chewing. His pale blue eyes brightened for a moment, then he said, "When I played Babe Ruth."

I was stunned, not knowing whether to believe him. My gut instinct told me it was true.

"Tell me about it."

Arthur leaned back in his chair. "I only played him once. August 1931. It was hotter 'n blazes that day. I was a rookie pitcher for the White Sox. Babe was nearing the end of his career. He had a reputation for boozin' and womanizin'. Damn near killed him. He couldn't even run the bases anymore. Anyway, I figured I had the advantage. Thought I

could get away with sneakin' a fast ball past him. Ha!..."
Arthur slapped his knee and grinned. "Soon as I heard the
crack of the bat, I knew it was over the fence. Learned one
thing, for sure. He didn't drink enough to slow him down."

I was sure the story had been told a hundred times
before. With passion and humor, Arthur talked on about the
early days of baseball, taking me back to a time I had only
read about. And, for a few glorious moments, I saw him
standing on the mound, throwing one more fast ball.

Eventually, his conversation returned to delusional
mutterings, and then he fell asleep. I sat with Arthur awhile
longer, knowing that my perception of old people had
changed forever. He had shown me that the heart and soul of
a young person lives on in the aging body.

I marveled at the realization that I had been witness to
the retelling of an historic event. It occurred to me that this
experience had only been possible because I had taken a
chance, a chance that just a few moments, a few kind words
could create a bridge across generations. And I wondered
about the day when no one would want to hear my stories any
more.

The Crisis of Aging

Ten centuries before the birth of Christ, Solomon, the
aged writer of Ecclesiastes, pondered the meaning of life and
death. He wrote, "To everything there is a season...A time to
be born and a time to die." Today, thousands of years later,
we continue to quote his famous words. This poetic phrase
holds a painful reminder of the brevity of our lives. While we

may think that Solomon had it "all together" and was comfortable with the reality of the life and death cycle, like us, he struggled with growing old. In Ecclesiastes 12, he refers to old age as the "dismal days."

> That is when the light of the sun, the moon, and the stars will grow dim for you, and the rain clouds will never pass away. Then your arms, that have protected you will tremble, and your legs, now strong, will grow weak. Your teeth will be too few to chew your food, and your eyes too dim to see clearly. Your ears will be deaf to the noise of the street. You will barely be able to hear the mill as it grinds or music as it plays, but even the song of a bird will wake you from your sleep...Your hair will turn white; you will hardly be able to drag yourself along and all desire will be gone.
>
> (Ecclesiastes 12: 1-5)
> Good News Bible

The decision to place a parent or loved one in a nursing home, causes us to consider the seasons of life. For a short time, we must turn away from our youth-centered existence to face the aging process and come to terms with our own mortality. For most of us this is an alarming thought. Our culture has such a strong bias toward youth that when we must deal with the realities of our decline or that of our parents, it comes as a shock to us.

Until this crisis, we are able to deceive ourselves into thinking that the relentless pursuit of youth will somehow indefinitely postpone our growing old. We focus on a Hollywood image of the beautiful life which we equate with happiness and immortality. Multi-million dollar industries are built around supporting this ideal. We purchase cosmetic surgeries, health and fitness programs, and age-defying products in our search for the elusive "fountain of youth." Author David Barash states it this way:

> To be human, it seems, is to be ambivalent. And perhaps no where is this ambivalence more clearly shown than in our attitudes toward aging. We seek to live long, yet we dread being old. [1]

What is interesting about our fixation with youth is its age-relatedness. In our early years, we mark the passing of time with birthdays that are viewed as major milestones. Beginning with the first year, there is almost an urgency to grow up. Birthdays continue to be a reason for celebration, until we reach adulthood. Then gradually, at some point in our twenties, the focus changes, and the approach to aging becomes humorous or grim. As we turn thirty, forty and fifty the tone of our greeting cards shifts to an "over-the-hill" mentality, and, for some, growing older becomes a reason to feel depressed.

The Last Thing We Talk About

Thus, we come to the subject of aging totally unprepared. We avoid thinking about it or talking about it. In a sense, it has become the last taboo. We are more willing to discuss the darker sides of our lives – addictions, sexual dysfunction, and family violence – because these are problems from which we hope to recover. We see old age as the beginning of the end.

This avoidance of aging and aging issues is so prevalent in our society that we have created a situation in which we stereotype the elderly. In our minds, growing old may be synonymous with frailty, dependence, loss of usefulness and diminished mental capacity. In fact, what we imagine about old age is more damaging to our thinking than the realities of growing old. We asked study participants: What do you fear about growing old?

> Alzheimer's, cancer, wrinkles, and no more physical beauty. It scares me. I'd rather die young while I still look youthful.   Kate...age 18

> Old age is depressing and lonely.   Cynthia...age 45

> I don't want to lose my freedom of movement and my health.   Felix...age 61

> I think growing old is hell. It's degrading, and we're not taught how to do it.   Jayne...age 34

In addition to our fears of growing old, we fear the loneliness and the dependency associated with aging. In our minds they are closely linked to each other. For some of the individuals, the subject of aging brought feelings of anger – feelings, perhaps derived from a sense of helplessness and the realization that despite the choices we make in life, all of us have the same destiny.

> When I seen an old person shuffling along with a cane or driving too slow in my lane of traffic, I become angry inside because I see my future.   Susan...age 50

False beliefs and fears about aging can have devastating consequences for society. The mistaken perception that aging is unnatural leads us to treat it like a cancer that must be eradicated, and this in turn fosters an avoidance of those we perceive to be old. Residents in nursing homes are often lonely and isolated because of our fears of old age. The growth of advocacy groups such as The National Center On Elder Abuse and the National Coalition for Nursing-Home Reform is the direct result of such discrimination against those who are alone, powerless, and under-represented.

Coming To Terms With Growing Old

Depending on one's perspective, old age may be the worst or the best of life. It is interesting to note that, even though all of our respondents feared what might happen when they become "old," they disagreed over the age at which "old" begins.

> My parents are old. Their hair is gray. They don't do as much as they use to. They go to bed early, their knees hurt. They're about 50.   Kate...age 18

> I don't think there's an age. It depends on your attitude and physical health.   Jayne...age 34

> None of us wants to be old. I think you're always twenty on the inside...until something reminds you, like when your body doesn't obey your mind.   Maria...age 73

While failing health is a factor in aging for some, greater numbers of people are living healthy, productive lives into their eighties, nineties and even beyond. There are many examples, but Mother Theresa was probably one of the most famous. She worked tirelessly among the poor in Calcutta, despite her advanced age and health problems. Comedian

George Burns continued in show business until his death at 100 years. And a best seller, *The Delaney Sisters' First 100 Years*, was written by two sisters when they were 103 and 104.

For some of the individuals we interviewed, growing old was not a negative.

> You're only as old as you feel. You have to tolerate what the Lord gives you. It's how you approach it, a matter of attitude. I think quality of life is most important.
> Jim...age 62
>
> I'd like to live to be 100, but not if I'm a burden to someone. Then I'd rather die.   Harold...age 93

As our Baby Boomer generation ages with its fixation on health and fitness, we can expect that greater numbers of us will live well into our eighties and nineties. It would appear that we strive to live forever, but are we willing to face the consequences of that goal? The end products may be declining health and dependence on others. We value youth because it offers time and hope. Old age holds no such promises. When youth disappears and health fails, our only hope is to look to eternity with God. Those who are wise enough to grasp this concept have less anxiety about the future. One nursing-home resident, who felt great satisfaction with her long life, expressed it this way:

> The advice I would give to people is to thank the Lord and take each day as it comes.   Anita...age 100

Like Solomon, we must accept old age as a season and trust that life and death are part of a greater plan designed for us by our Heavenly Father.

I have been young
and now I am old.
And in all my years
I have never seen
the Lord forsake a man
who loves him.

(Psalm 37:25)
Living Bible

Suggestions for Families

As a society, we attempt to protect ourselves from the realities of aging because of our own fears about growing old. We focus on youth so that old age won't happen to us. As a result, the needs of the frail elderly and the issues that affect their care are often overlooked. This lack of sensitivity will have its impact on our lives and those of future generations. Our involvement in the care and concerns of our elders will set the example of how our children will care for us in the future.

Encourage your children to learn more about their elderly relatives and neighbors by having a celebration of age. Plan a birthday party for an older person. Focus on a theme, such as the Roaring Twenties or any historic event that was significant in his or her early years. The results will enrich the lives of all involved.

If your children don't have grandparents or their grandparents live far away, adopt some. Visit elderly neighbors or friends. Invite them to celebrate holidays with you.

Volunteer at a local nursing home, group home or assisted living facility. There is always something you can do to help.

Encourage elders to talk about their lives. Record Dad's favorite stories on tape. Work on your family tree together.

Additional Resources

Learn to Grow Old, Paul Tournier, Westminster John Knox Press, 1991.

Reflections on Aging: A Spiritual Guide, Leo E. Missinne, Liguori Publications, 1990.

Fifty To Forever, Hugh Downs, Thomas Nelson, 1994.

CHAPTER THREE

The
Nursing-Home
Decision

And now, in my old age,
don't set me aside.
Don't forsake me now when my
strength is failing.

(Psalm 71:9)
Living Bible

Mama

Mama always said she never wanted to go to a nursing home, that she'd rather be dead. It wasn't that she made me promise or anything, but she made it clear she didn't want to go.

Mama was the strong and independent type. She felt good about "doing for others." She was a nurse in the old-fashioned sense of the word, and a good one. There always seemed to be people at our door needing insulin injections, or a dressing changed, maybe a few days of post-operative care. Our house often smelled of rubbing alcohol. In the summer, neighbors would bring sweaty children with skinned knees or bee stings to ask Mama if she thought they should call the doctor. Mama loved to be needed, and no one was ever turned away.

We were very close, Mama and I. I remember a game we would play when she got sick. I got to be the nurse and bring her a drink of water. Sometimes she'd let me wear her starched nurse's cap that was kept safe under her sweaters in the bottom drawer of her upright dresser. It made me feel very special. When I grew up and got married, the relationship continued. We'd visit or talk on the phone every day. We could talk about anything, just like best friends. I always knew that I would take care of Mama, if I had to.

When my grandparents got old, they came to live in our house. The pipe stand and leather chair were moved out of Papa's den, and beds were moved in. A nursing home wasn't even considered.

Mama said, "Nursing homes are terrible places," even though she and Papa knew someone who lived at the Lutheran Home and liked it.

But Papa said, "You can trust the Lutherans, but you have to turn your money over to them."

Grandpa died suddenly. A few months later, Grandma got cancer. I watched Mama take care of her, just like she was in the hospital. The doctor would come to give his orders, and she would follow them to the letter. Grandma often required her attention day and night, especially at the end. I never once heard Mama complain.

Years later, when Mama had a mild stroke, I planned to do the same. I fussed over fixing up the spare room to make her welcome. I planned how I would work her into my busy schedule and care for the children at the same time, just as she had done. The day of her arrival, I hurried to make her bed, folding up the bottom corners, hospital style, as she had taught me. I brushed my hands over the cool sheets to make them smooth. The phone rang. Mama was back in the hospital with a massive stroke. I laid down on the bed and cried. I would not be able to care for her at home.

I'll never forget the moment we told her about the nursing home. Mama's eyes widened, then she turned her face away from me. After that, she never spoke again.

At first, I went to visit often. I would find her sitting up in bed looking out the window. But, when Mama heard my voice, she would shut her eyes and refuse to acknowledge me. Maybe it was anger that I had not taken her home. Maybe it was the humiliation of her helplessness.

The last five months of her life Mama and I would play a game. I would visit. Mama would shut her eyes. I would tell her I loved her, kiss her forehead and leave. Mama never wanted to go to a nursing home.

The Sandwich Generation

The aging of America is a medical success story of the 20th century. Lower infant mortality rates and the ability to effectively fight many diseases have made it possible for a person born since the 1950s to live almost twice as many years as his grandparents. This trend has resulted in a rapidly growing population of individuals over age sixty-five. While it is our desire to live longer and more productive lives, these changes have brought about a complex set of problems for our society. A new question must now be answered, "How do we care for the increasing numbers of people who, because of age, have become dependent on others for care?"

As our population continues to age, and older and older children care for very elderly parents, the problem will become even more complicated. Individuals who are in their seventies and eighties are now caring for parents who are in their nineties and one hundreds. Often these aged "children" have health problems or financial difficulties. In such cases, the responsibility for both parents and grandparents may transfer to the third generation, and these individuals, who are in their forties or fifties, may be raising young children of their own.

Dealing with parents who grow old and require our help in greater amounts of time and energy puts us in direct conflict with our own priorities. On the one hand, mom may need care and supervision, and on the other, we are sandwiched between generations with responsibilities to our own family, our career and even to ourselves. The sacrifice may be too great, leaving us angry and exhausted.

> I just finished raising my own kids, and now I'm starting all over again, taking care of my parents.   Dora...age 57

Family Traditions And Eldercare

How individual families approach the solution to eldercare is influenced by many factors. Beliefs about family responsibility and cultural traditions play an important part in this decision. For some elderly individuals, being cared for by family is an expected benefit of growing old. Anything less is considered to be an avoidance of one's responsibilities. When we asked nursing-home residents about their feelings toward institutional living, some expressed resentment that the younger generation does not do its part.

> In my day, it was a disgrace to send someone to a nursing home. It meant you didn't care much for your family.   Sherman...age 93

Individuals raised in an environment that supported the position of "caring for your own" may have strong convictions about their responsibilities and feel that nursing homes represent an abandonment of their obligations. Some of these beliefs reflect family tradition, others are cultural in origin.

My grandparents lived with us until they died. After
that, one of my great aunts came to stay with us for
terminal care. I was only eighteen. I remember changing
her diapers. It was what our family did.   Karen...age 54

In the Hispanic community, we keep our people at
home. It's hard, but they are happier. At least you know
what you give them. A stranger, like a nurse or a
volunteer, doesn't have the same feelings as a daughter
or son. There are young people, children who are
bedridden. Why should it be different if you are older?
Maria...age 72

In addition to the influences of family example and
cultural traditions, our beliefs about caring for elders are also
shaped by the views we hold toward institutional care. The
collective attitudes of our elders, society and the media, along
with negative personal experiences, can provide a strong bias
against nursing homes.

The Stigma Of Nursing Homes

The term "nursing home" has a long history of
negative associations dating back to the early part of this
century. At that time, the elderly were institutionalized with
the mentally ill, mentally handicapped and indigents in such
places as county hospitals and poor houses. Persons who had
to go to the poor house were identified by their economic
misfortune or were assumed to have no family who could take
care of them, a stigma that exists today. As nursing homes
developed and took over the function of care for elderly and
disabled individuals, the negative reputation continued.

Unfortunately, the conditions in both state and private institutions were appalling and remained unchanged until the 1970s.

Nursing-home reform movements during the 1980s resulted in new state and federal laws that have made the long-term care industry one of the most highly regulated in the United States. In 1987, the federal government enacted legislation called the Omnibus Budget Reconciliation Act (OBRA). The emphasis of OBRA is on protecting residents' rights and ensuring quality care to all individuals in nursing facilities. Quality care, as defined by OBRA, must promote an individual resident's highest level of functioning, thus reducing the physical and mental decline often associated with living in a nursing home.

These changes have brought about a new emphasis on rehabilitation in the long-term care setting, a benefit to both residents and facilities. By increasing the focus on therapy services provided to residents under Medicare, many individuals are able to return home or move to a less restrictive environment, such as assisted living or group homes. The benefit to facilities is that they can capture the more lucrative Medicare dollar by providing these services and promoting shorter stays and rehabilitation.

The emphasis, in long-term care, is to down play the idea that individuals in nursing homes are aging. The focus is on the potential for rehabilitation and a return to community living. For many families this creates hope that their parent will get well, or at least there will be a delay of the unavoidable. In reality, the majority of residents will find that the front door of a nursing home swings in only one direction. Most will call this "home" for the rest of their days.

The long-term care industry is making an attempt to change the image of eldercare. Facilities have stopped calling themselves nursing homes and, instead, refer to their institutions as health-care centers, subacute units or transitional care. It has been predicted that short-term facilities are the future, and nursing homes, as we know them today, will gradually disappear.

When a family tours a nursing home, they may be surprised to learn that it is very different from what they expected to find. Many of the newer facilities are designed to look like luxury apartments with home-style furnishings and beautifully decorated dining and lounge areas. These more expensive accommodations are intended to appeal to the younger generations, who shop for a facility and choose placement for their family members.

While state and federal regulations have made a significant impact on the quality of eldercare, these changes have not had a notable effect on public opinion. Problems in nursing homes still exist. Because of bad publicity, very few people are aware of the positive changes. The end result is that many people continue to have a biased view of what goes on inside the confines of these institutions. When we interviewed participants about their feelings toward nursing homes, all responded with negative comments.

> Hospital beds, wheelchairs, that's what I think of.
> Carol...age 42

> An old smell...urine, perspiration, with a cover-up of
> vanilla musk in the air.   Kate...age 18

I think the stories are true. There's a lot of abuse. When my dad was in one, they would leave people in wet diapers and handcuff them to their beds.   Joan...age 48

I told my wife that if I ever get to the point where I have to go in a nursing home, I'll stick my head in the oven. Dick...age 67

One participant even referred to it as a "loony bin," associating the behaviors of dementia with mental illness. Still another stated that going to a nursing home meant you were crazy.

Today, the media and the public in general continue to emphasize the negative side of long-term care. We do such a great job of bad mouthing nursing homes that, when it's time to make a decision, we feel immense guilt. We set up expectations that box us into a corner. I don't want to go. I don't want my parents to go. They shouldn't go. But the reality is...will we be able or willing to care for them at home?

The Nursing-home Decision

Perhaps the need for long-term care would be easier for us to accept if we all prepared for the end of life by giving it as much thought as we do in preparing for the beginning. Again, our focus is on youth. The birth of a baby, how we raise our children, education and career advancement are things we plan for in our earlier years. Few individuals have the foresight to select retirement facilities that will care for them if they become incapacitated. If this decision were discussed ahead of time, families could be spared the stress of making the nursing-home decision in a crisis.

It would be easier if they would choose to go. Camilla...age 50

> I always tell my kids, "Put me in a nursing home if I get
> so you can't take care of me." I'm sure that when the
> time comes, they may still feel guilt, but I told them to
> do it. Cynthia...age 45

Most families don't talk about long-term care because
it is too difficult to face the thought of growing old. By
avoiding the subject, we may fool ourselves into thinking the
decision will never have to be made.

> My mother and I think the same way about nursing
> homes. We don't like them, but I've never brought it up
> with my kids.   Joan...age 49

Currently, only five percent of Americans over the age
of sixty-five require institutional care. The remainder live out
their lives at home or with family members. "It is simply not
true that large numbers of older people are 'dumped' into
nursing homes by uncaring offspring. This is one of the myths
that no amount of data can dislodge from the public mind.
Most institutional placement occurs after all other alternatives
have been tried, and particularly after a major health setback
to the older person or some change in the ability of adult
children to provide care." [1]

Despite our desire to keep loved ones in the
community, we may encounter difficulties in caring for them
at home. The decision to place often results in a tremendous
amount of guilt. It raises the question of whether our parents
spent that amount of time for us when we needed them.

> It was real hard to place my mother. My brother and I
> both felt we were letting her down. I kept thinking,
> "Maybe if I had kept her with us longer, the progression

of the illness (Alzheimer's) may have slowed down...maybe if she had been with people she loved." I still feel guilty. I think, "No matter what had been wrong with me, she would have taken care of me."
Mary...age 54

Unfortunately, most families approach the nursing-home decision in a crisis. Their loved ones may suddenly need care, due to physical or mental decline, and there is no other choice but to protect them.

I knew it was time to place my mother the day she burned up a pan of cookies. I was terrified that she would hurt herself.   Mary...age 54

It was the 5th of November. I got a call from the police. A neighbor found my mother in her backyard without a coat or scarf on. She was all bruised from falling. After that, we took her home with us, but she kept us up all night. All of us had jobs."   Maryanne...46

Whatever the crisis, if we are unwilling or unable to meet the needs of our aging family members, we must face the alternative, placing them in the care of strangers.

"I lived with my daughter. I became too much work for her. She had a job. Every time she wanted to go some place, she had to get a babysitter for me and that wasn't always easy. She talked to me, explaining that it was too hard. I told her to do it quickly."   Mae...87

Suggestions for Families

The best time to make a decision about eldercare is long before the need arises. The worst time is in a crisis. If parents and children or grandchildren are able to have open discussions about their wishes regarding eldercare options, it eases the burden of the individual who must make the decision about placement.

Because of negative attitudes about nursing homes, many elders are unwilling to discuss what might happen to them if they need care in the future. One of the best ways to open a discussion with your family members is to begin talking about what you want for yourself.

All family members should have a power of attorney for health care. This is a document that allows each individual to state his or her wishes regarding end-of-life decisions and nursing-home placement. The power of attorney for health care also appoints another person as a decision-maker in the event that the individual making the document becomes incapacitated and unable to make his or her wishes known. Power of attorney for health care documents can be obtained from health care providers, such as hospitals and nursing homes or from individual state departments of health and human services.

Be informed about eldercare options in your community. Tour facilities before you need to place someone. Ask for recommendations from friends, your local church or your family physician. There are also many good resources available to help you choose the best possible facility.

Additional Resources

Choosing a Nursing Home, Seth B. Goldsmith, Prentice Hall, 1990.

How To Care For Aging Parents, Virginia Morris, Workman Publishing, 1996.

Fifty To Forever, Hugh Downs, Thomas Nelson, 1994.

CHAPTER FOUR

How Do I Tell My Father He Has To Stay?

Anyone who neglects to care for family members in need repudiates the faith. That's worse than refusing to believe in the first place.

(1 Timothy 5:8)
The Message

Jake

Everyone who lives here would rather be home. There ain't no place like home. Always a few residents hanging around the front door waitin' for their kinfolk or tryin' to get out. That's why we got them door alarms.

I've been housekeepin' in this nursin' home for twenty-six years now, guess you'd say I'm an old timer. Started out in the kitchen, then I got this here promotion. The boss always says, "Myra, you're a fine example of a dedicated employee." Even got awards, I did.

You get to know the residents and their kin real good when you clean up after 'em every day. You do a good job and they trust you with their personal things, get to tellin' you about their families and all. I seen a lot of things in my time and heard a lot of secrets, too.

The saddest thing I ever seen was Jake. He come here from the farm. Born and raised there, his cousin told me. He was kinda ornery, talked rude-like to his family, what family he had. Never married. The cousin and his wife done the best they could by him. Tried to help him out at home, but he was durn stubborn, wouldn't do nothin' but sit in his chair by the TV day and night. Finally got so sick the county worker came and got him, brought him here cause he was neglectin' hisself.

They said old Jake had forty-three cats in his house. Can you imagine that? Boy, oh boy, glad I wasn't cleanin up after them cats. Of course, it was me who cleaned up his stuff once he got here. I done a real fine job, too. They had to throw out the clothes he come in. Whew, that room did smell like a cat box.

His family went and bought him all bran' new clothes. They was right about him bein' ornery. Why he wouldn't even try 'em on, at first. I said to him, "Jake, you'd look mighty fine in that there red plaid shirt your cousin buyed ya." One mornin' there he was a-showin' hisself off to me, sportin' that red shirt an' a new pair of trousers. I told him he looked like a youngun' goin' a-courtin'. Only time I ever did see him smile.

Nope, Jake never did appreciate nuthin' a body did for him. Yes siree, that man could swear a streak. He'd just cuss out his cousin every chance he got. I'd try to tell him, "Now Jake, you treat your kinfolk nice, they's all you have." But it didn't seem to matter much. He was already gone in the head by the time he come to this place.

Every day he'd ask to use the phone, over and over again, maybe ten, fifteen times, he'd be pesterin' me or the nurse to call his cousin. Once in a while he'd call a neighbor. It didn't matter who answered. The message was always the same. "This here's Jake. You'all come git me. I wanna go home."

Then, when they'd come to visit, he'd cuss at 'em some more for bringin' him here. Sometimes he'd refuse to talk. Poor old Jake, he just didn't understand.

I remember one time, his cousin got so mad I heard him shout. "Face it Jake, this is the end of the line! You're here to die." I thought that was awful mean, him bein' demented and all. I told the social worker, I did.

Jake never stopped makin' those calls 'till just before the end. After awhile, the family started lyin' to him, and that's a fact. I heard 'em. Just to stop the pesterin', they'd tell him they was comin' in the afternoon to pick him up. That old

Jake, he'd put on his hat and coat and sit by the front door, wouldn't eat lunch or anything 'cause he didn't want to miss 'em.

Yup, we all want to go home, but some just don't understand they're here to stay.

Our Responsibility To Family

We learn to believe through faith and custom that families should care for their own. Scripture provides us with many examples of how God expects us to care for family members. Perhaps the most familiar of these is the fourth commandment. In Exodus 20:12, we are told, "Honor your father and mother." Both the Old and New Testaments have directives about our responsibilities toward parents, widows, orphans, and the poor. For those of us who wish to please God, caring for family members may be viewed as a rule of our faith.

To make a decision that contradicts these beliefs can create emotional conflict and guilt. Placement is certainly not what we would want for ourselves, and at our deepest level of feeling, we know that how and where we spend the rest of our lives is not a choice that should be made by others.

The Good Old Days

The problem of eldercare has been an issue in society since the beginning of time. Every culture had its own unique way of dealing with elderly people who, because of age, were no longer making a significant contribution to society. Some cultures revered their aged members, caring for them with great compassion. Some were guilty of neglect, abandonment and even murder.

We would like to think that "in the good old days" (those years our parents and grandparents remember fondly), extended families lived together in harmony under one roof, each making a contribution to the group as a whole. Our elders may have cited numerous examples from past generations, where grandma and grandpa or aunts and uncles lived in multi-generational households. Whether these situations were always as perfect and harmonious as they have been remembered could be questioned. For some they were workable and satisfying arrangements that made economic sense at the time.

Quite often, there are families who have been able to work out similar situations, caring for parents or grandparents because of available time, space or finances. But the truth is that yesterday's solutions to eldercare are not always practical or appropriate for the present.

As we approach the end of the 20th century, advances in health and medicine have given new meaning to the concept of "taking care of your own." In the late 1800s, for example, the average life expectancy was about forty-six years. In the last 100 years, it has nearly doubled. The figures for 1995 are seventy-two years for a man and seventy-nine years for a woman. Currently, in the United States, there are 33 million people over the age of sixty-five and nearly 3.5 million over the age of eighty-five. "In this century, the rate of growth of the elderly population (persons 65 years old and over) has greatly exceeded the growth rate of the population of the country as a whole." [1]

Children who are past retirement age are now taking care of parents who are eighty to one hundred, and these *oldest of the old* often need skilled nursing care and around-the-clock supervision.

> My mother lived with me until she was ninety-eight.
> Then she lost her vision, and I just couldn't take care of
> her any more.   Frances...age 82

The composition of our population has changed so significantly that we must review our thinking about eldercare. It is no longer practical to make decisions based only on prior beliefs or experiences, and we must be careful not to judge ourselves or others too harshly for making the decision to place someone in a nursing facility. The solutions we seek today must fit the problems of an aging population. So, while we may feel tremendous guilt for placing a loved one in an institution, we must be realistic in the ability of family members or friends to provide care.

No Easy Answers

It is most often, an adult child who comes to the nursing home to place a parent. Sometimes, it is a spouse or a grandchild. Occasionally, a more distant relative or friend has taken on this role. For anyone who must make the nursing-home decision on behalf of another person, this is an unpleasant, and often painful, task.

> When I made the decision to place Joe, he was in such
> bad shape, mentally and physically. I felt bad. I still feel
> bad. My great regret is that he has never asked, "How
> did I get here?" Which makes me think, "He doesn't
> want to know."   Dorothy...age 58

The initial tour of a facility is very difficult for most family members. Even individuals who are convinced that they have made the only possible choice come to the admission process with fears and uncertainty, not to mention negative feelings, about nursing homes in general. Families admit their uneasiness and dislike for what they are about to do. Some have great difficulty just being in the building. One woman who was about to place her mother, burst into tears as she walked through a visiting area.

> My mother always said there was a purpose to everything, but I don't see a purpose to living like this. Carla...age 49

When it is a spouse or elderly "child" who must make the nursing-home decision, the placement process becomes even more complicated. Frequently, individuals who place a loved one are themselves senior citizens and may have their own physical and mental limitations due to age. In this instance, the older decision-makers are forced to deal with a health care system that overwhelms them by it complexity.

> When I had to place my husband, I didn't know anything about the system. There were so many papers to sign, things I didn't understand. I don't think they did a good job of explaining things to me. I felt I was at their mercy. Lonnie...age 75

Whatever the age or circumstances of the people involved, someone is responsible for making the nursing-home decision. The ability to make this choice effectively is influenced by many factors: beliefs about family, the safety and well-being of the individual who needs care, and the willingness and competence of others to provide the care needed at home.

Ideally, the person who needs placement should be able to say, "I know that I can no longer care for myself and choose to go to a nursing home." When this happens, there is a tremendous amount of relief for family and friends because they are excused from doing the difficult task.

More frequently, family members and the person needing care make the decision together. A crisis, such as illness or injury, may precipitate the need for twenty-four-hour medical care or a more supervised environment. Often, the physician insists on placement for the safety and well being of the individual. If the elderly person understands this, he may not want to be a burden to his family and will agree to placement. Even though many older persons fear nursing homes, they may greatly respect the advice of their family doctor and never think to question his authority. When the physician recommends placement, and the family and resident are able to agree with his advice, this removes the blame from family members and allows the persons involved to grieve the loss together.

Facing The Facts

The real difficulty comes when the individual is no longer able to make decisions that are in his own best interest. Unless a surrogate decision-maker has been appointed through power of attorney for health care or guardianship, the person needing care must agree to placement and, in effect, sign himself into a facility. If this individual has been negative about nursing homes and has expressed, to his family and friends that he will *never* go to one, the problem can be stressful for everyone involved.

Each family will handle this situation differently. Some children are able to assume the leadership position without difficulty. In this case, the parent looks to the child for advice and accepts the reversal of roles.

> I lived in Virginia. My daughter lives here. She made the decision. I was very annoyed at the time, but the more I thought about it, well, she has two teenagers, and having an old lady in the house is not the ideal situation. Bertha...age 90

Some families choose to avoid the truth. They keep saying, "When you get better or stronger, you'll go home." They put off telling their parent because they fear the rejection or anger of the person they must place.

> My husband asks and asks to go home. He wants to see the flowers in his garden before winter comes, but we're afraid we won't be able to get him to come back here. Sarah...age 85

When the nursing-home resident is not told by his family that he has to stay, or if he forgets that they have told him, he looks to the staff for a response. If his questions are left unanswered, he may become depressed and angry.

> All my life I took care of my children, and when they worked, I took care of their children. When my mother and father got old, I took them in, too. Now I need someone to take care of me, and no one has the time. They just put me in a place like this and forget about me." Lydia...age 93

Within the framework of an aging population, we are called to minister to those in need. In the face of change, we must expand our thinking and ask new questions about our obligations to those we love. For example, instead of looking at placement as abandonment, are we able to broaden our perspective of what it means to care for our own? Is it possible to extend our personal "care zone"? In what ways can we remain involved after placement, and perhaps even manage the care-giving process? By asking better questions, we learn to come to terms with what we perceive to be our responsibility. In this way we can be at peace with our decisions.

Lord, when doubts fill my mind,
when my heart is in turmoil,
quiet me and give me
renewed hope and cheer.

(Psalm 94:19)
Living Bible

Suggestions for Families

The transition from home to nursing home can be less traumatic when families continue to spend time together. If your parent or loved one is angry about placement, don't abandon him. Continue to be supportive by visiting and getting involved in the activities of his new living arrangement.

If possible, try to continue some of the rituals you shared as a family. One daughter had tea with her mother every Wednesday afternoon. She brought two place settings of her mother's favorite china, a pretty tablecloth, cookies and coffee.

Take your parent out for a drive or home for holiday visits if his or her condition permits. Have the family gather together at the facility for special occasions, such as football games, birthdays and other events.

Encourage your parents to make as many decisions as possible regarding their new environment. Support them in issues, such as how they want their personal care done, what clothes they would like to wear and their food preferences.

Additional Resources

The Long-Term Care Family Manual, MaryLou Hughes, Professional Printing & Publishing, Inc. 1995.

CHAPTER FIVE

For One Room Only

*My years are passing now and
I walk the road of no return.*

(Job 16:22)
Good News Bible

Patsy

So you want to interview me, do you? What could I possibly tell you? I'm ninety years old. I've lived a good life. I really have no regrets. I'm ready to go. Every night before I go to sleep, I say, "God take me," but he never does.

I was a nurse, you know. Back then, we didn't sit and do paperwork like they do now. Why, then a chart was a board that you hung on the end of the bed, not big thick folders. Is it the government that makes them write all that stuff?

I worked at Presbyterian Hospital in New York City. Back in my day, you had thirty-four patients on one ward, and you took care of all of them. I remember one poor soul who was going upstairs for surgery. The head nurse told me to get a specimen from this young fella. She was a nasty old bat; we were all afraid of her, called her Nurse Ratchet. Well, anyway, I sang, I danced, I ran water, but the poor guy just couldn't give. So I did it for him. Can you imagine that? He could have died, but everything turned out all right, thank God. Did I tell you I was a nurse? Oh yes, of course I did. Why am I so forgetful, dear? Do you think it's my age?

Did I tell you how I met my husband? My friends and I always ate lunch at this little cafe called The Greasy Spoon. We were sitting at the counter, and a beggar walked in off the street selling violets, like they do. Well, anyway, this very handsome man, who was sitting a few seats down from me, bought a bunch of violets, put them in his water glass, pushed it in front of me, and introduced himself.

He said he wanted to go to a party out on Long Island, but he didn't have a car. I had just bought a 1934 Ford Roadster, paid $625 for it, so I loaned him my keys. My friends said, "You're crazy, Patsy, you'll never see that man or your car again." But a couple of days later, he brought it back. We were married on New Year's Day. He was a wonderful man, always remembered to buy me violets. He was a lawyer for the *New York Herald Tribune*, a brilliant man. That's his picture there on the wall. He's gone many years now. We had a wonderful life. I have no regrets. And there's a picture of our house in Connecticut with my husband and I standing out front. That picture over there is Spokey, our Yorkshire terrier; actually he's a mixture, Heinz 57 variety, but we loved him.

Are you the one that helped me hang all my pictures? I want to thank you. They mean so much to me. After all, this is everything I have left, right here in this room. Actually, this half is my side of the room. My roommate, she's a little forgetful, has a tendency to steal things, you know. Not that she means to, poor dear, but she's a bit confused. Takes my teddy bear and puts it on her bed. I like to sleep with my teddy bear. You probably think I'm an old fool doing something like that.

What was it you asked me, dear? Oh yes, what was the most exciting thing that ever happened to me? Well, I wouldn't call it exciting, but it really was very sad. Those poor young captains, who were burned in the crash of the Hindenburg, we took care of them at Presbyterian Hospital. We didn't have plastic surgery back then. Nowadays, you walk in the doctor's office and pick out a face. They can make you look whatever way you want. But, we couldn't do that then. They were so horribly burned and such handsome young men, too.

Well, anyway, I escorted them back to Germany on the Europa. We changed their dressings every two hours. After that, I lived in Europe for two years, traveled around at the expense of the German government. They were grateful for the care I had given the captains. I even saw Austria, where the *Sound of Music* was made. It's always been my favorite movie.

Is there anything else you wanted to know, dear? I've really not much to tell you. I'm getting very tired and would like to lie down. I'll be ninety-one soon. Did I tell you that? Tell me, what earthly good am I still living at this age? I'm ready. Teddy and I will go to bed and ask God one more time.

A Lifetime Of Losses

The tragedy of long-term placement is that it separates an individual from the familiar. For most of us, life begins surrounded by ritual and community. Family and friends rejoice at the birth of a new baby. As the child grows, there is a continued observance of significant days in that individual's life. Occasions such as: Baptism, birthdays, graduations, marriage and anniversaries are all reasons to celebrate. Even in death, there is a sense of belonging. We gather to remember and mourn the life that has passed. But, as author Renee Rose Shield observes, the "entrance to the nursing home (is) a rite of passage with few, if any, rituals. The entrance is lonely, accomplished primarily by a series of leave-takings from a past life." [1]

The losses that an individual suffers on admission to a nursing home are profound and irreversible. Whether a person has lived in his own home or with family members, there is an accumulation of possessions and a network of relationships that have, over time, reinforced one's sense of belonging. To leave these behind is a lonely transition. Throughout our lifetime, we establish homes, build careers, accumulate possessions and nurture relationships. We never imagine that some day these will all be taken away from us – that we cannot keep, and will never get back, what we have struggled so hard to gain. Home, family, friends, possessions; these are the very things that we use to define who we really are. When they are gone, we might ask, "What is left?" One elderly woman, unhappy about living with her grandchildren, expressed her frustration with giving up the things she owned.

> Look what has happened to me. I've worked hard all my
> life and now, everything I own is in one room!
> Edna...age 79

How residents cope with the transition from home to nursing home, falls into three general categories. For some there is a denial. These individuals passively ignore the changes that have taken place in their lives, choosing not to discuss the hurt or disappointment that is a natural result of the losses they have experienced. They may withdraw from social relationships and are more likely to express hopelessness or become depressed, even to the extent that they may give up on life and will themselves to die soon after admission.

The second group of residents reacts to placement with anger. This may be directed toward caregivers or family members in the form of outbursts of temper or criticism. The purpose is to punish those individuals that they feel are responsible for their losses. These individuals alienate family and friends and, as a result, create more losses because loved ones tend to stay away.

The third group of residents are those who are accepting of loss. They are able to talk about their feelings and work through the grief of life changes. Their sadness is based in the reality that nothing remains the same, yet they can adjust and find peace and joy in any situation.

> What would I say to someone about living in a nursing home? I'd tell them to accept their lives, not fight it. It's not going to get you anywhere, just make it more difficult for you.   Patsy...age 90

Saying Good-bye To The Past

To fully understand the impact of the passage from home to a nursing home, we asked our focus groups to make a list of things they valued most in their lives. For younger generations, this was a typical response:

> My husband and children, listening to my daughter play the piano, the flower garden, a bird house outside my kitchen window, our home, my birthstone ring, friends, job, our dog Missy, my hobbies, good health.
> Kathy...age 39

After they had completed their lists, we asked them to begin crossing off the items they could not take with them to a nursing home. When asked to read the new list, group members were shocked and saddened.

I couldn't take any of these things, even my favorite
possession. It's a little green vase with a squirrel on it
that belonged to my grandmother. Why, it would be
stolen!   Mary...age 47

Living in a nursing home means losing all your
property. Maybe it's just a candlestick that you want to
keep, but you can't have it.   Kate...age 18

When we questioned nursing-home residents about the
things they valued, their answers were very different from the
younger generations. Not one person mentioned possessions
or indicated that they grieved the loss of "things."

What I value the most is family, memories and
friendship. It was different when I was younger. I valued
what appealed to me at the time.   Patsy...age 90

In general, we found that individuals in the community
who had not experienced the losses associated with living in a
nursing home, were more likely to value the touchable
"things" of life with which they surrounded themselves.
Residents in nursing facilities were more inclined to cherish
the intangibles, such as relationships. Despite these
differences, both groups had one primary concern that
connected them to each other. They both valued their
independence.

Freedom: The Greatest Loss

It is interesting to note that individuals surveyed were
concerned most with the loss of freedom that would take
place if they had to live in a nursing home. This fear was
expressed by residents, family members and caregivers. All
participants cherished their freedom above all other things.

> What do I think it's like to live in nursing home? Loss of independence, loss of decision making. It can be depressing, depending on where you are.   Judy...age 38

The struggle to become independent starts at birth and traditionally culminates in our leaving home as young adults. Throughout our lives, we battle with our parents and those in authority, for control over the decisions that affect us and are in conflict with our wishes. The desire for freedom is an innate yearning that enables us to care for ourselves, to create families of our own and to survive in a hostile world. Freedom and independence are fundamental to our existence. To lose them is, perhaps, the most devastating of experiences.

> My definition of being old is not being able to do what you want.   Lynette...age 43

> I had to give up my car and my independence. Lorraine...age 84

> I miss just going to the store and buying something, or eating at my favorite restaurant.   Bernice...73

Despite significant loss and change, we found an incredible resilience among the elderly in nursing homes. Those who survived the transition all agreed that the adjustment had been difficult, that they would rather be home. Those who succeeded in coping considered it a matter of attitude.

Perhaps the most touching statement came from Bernice who had lived in a facility for three years. She shared a small room with another resident who was somewhat confused. The room was crowded with remnants of their lives: a favorite dresser, family pictures, a couple of television sets, cards and letters from friends, along with the necessary wheelchairs and walkers. There was a sense of sadness to her losses, but for Bernice, life still held challenges, and acceptance meant reaching out to others.

> It's very difficult when you've lived by yourself, and now you can't make your own decisions anymore. You have to go with the flow here. You have to give up a lot of your own personality. But, you can take a look at the people around you and see what you can do for them. Bernice...age 92

Suggestions for Families

The loss of home and possessions can be devastating for the elderly resident who moves into a long-term care facility. If possible, allow your parents or loved ones to be involved in choosing which things they will take with them and which they will give away. Make the new environment as home-like as possible. Bring along favorite pictures, a chair or end table, a dresser, if space permits. Even a special afghan can be comforting and will help residents identify the new room as their space.

Reminiscing is a valuable tool for helping our elders make the transition from home to nursing home. It encourages them to review their life accomplishments, it helps to bridge the gap between generations and it has historical significance. Everyone has a story to tell. Remember Alex Haley's *Roots*? Your family may be next. Encourage reminiscence by talking about famous events in history. Read the newspaper together, and ask your elders how things were different or similar in their day.

Additional Resources

Remembering Your Story, Richard L. Morgan, Upper Room Books, 1996. A guide for assisting and encouraging elders to reminisce about their lives.

First Writes, Forty Writing Exercises For Older Adults, Margaret Gulsvig, BiFokal Productions, 809 Williamson St. Madison, WI 53703 (608-251-2818). Also available through libraries.

CHAPTER SIX

Those Left Behind

We are sick
at our very hearts
and can hardly
see through our tears.

(Lamentations 5:17)
Good News Bible

David

They sat together at the window of his room, waiting for the sun to set. Beth sipped "visitors only" coffee from a plastic mug and wished she could warm herself against David's body, but the steel frame of a wheelchair separated them. She considered the narrow bed where they could lie together in the fading light, nestled in each other's arms. The thought of someone finding them embarrassed her.

The room was small, but it had a west window. Beth had insisted on a west window when she brought him here. It was the least she could do. They loved to watch the sunsets together. For sixteen years this had been their special time, a break from the frenzy of work and children, a half-hour for coffee and intimate conversation. Now, it was a moment of awkward silence.

The mug was cool and safe to offer him. She held it to David's lips, pressing her napkin under his chin. He took little sips, closed his mouth too soon and made a mess. Beth set the coffee aside and wiped his face.

Few words passed between them anymore. The complexities of language were lost to him, and Beth, tired of one-sided conversations, no longer tried to pretend everything was the same. Sometimes David could manage to echo, "Hello sweetheart," if she said it first. Had it been months or years since they had really talked? Beth couldn't remember.

She twisted the gold band on her finger. In sickness and in health was their promise. He was forty-eight when he placed it there. She was thirty-two.

"Would he notice if I took it off?" she wondered.

Her solitary life had created opportunities and, more recently, the need to be with someone else. David's absence had left an emptiness that no amount of work or her love for their children could ever fill. Without him she felt so alone. Beth needed the warmth of a loving man, but never at sunset. This would always be their special time.

Beth turned on the radio to fill the void. "Rogers and Hammerstein, dear. Our favorite." Softly, she began to sing along.

> Hello, young lovers, wherever you are.
> I hope your troubles are few.

"Do you remember, David? We saw Yul Brynner on stage. It was the night you proposed."

David opened his mouth, but no words formed. Gently, she wiped spittle from his chin with her fingers.

> Be brave, young lovers,
> and follow your star.

"You swept me off my feet, darling. We were so much in love."

It didn't matter, then, that he was older. It mattered now. She was angry that he was leaving her. Alzheimer's was an unfair sentence for the father of young children, her lover, her friend.

> Cling very close to each other tonight.
> I've been in love, like you.

Beth lifted David's hands in both of hers and pressed her lips to his fingers. His eyes glistened with a hint of tears. Her body ached for the touch of his.

> Don't cry, young lovers,
> Whatever you do.
> Don't cry because I'm alone.
> All of my memories
> Are happy tonight.
> I've had a love of my own.

Changing Relationships

Loved ones who participate in the move from home to nursing home will experience their own losses as a result of this transition. When an older person can no longer live independently due to physical or mental decline, we must face the fact that he or she has changed in some way. These changes, whether sudden or gradual, cause a significant alteration of family life. If a parent or spouse is not the person he or she used to be, there is an interruption of familiar relationships and a shift in the roles we play. We feel sad because we mourn the loss of companionship and the individual's rightful place in our lives. For many, the grieving starts here.

> "My mother had many small strokes. It was like losing a part of her a little at a time."   Norma...62

Although sadness is the most common emotion that families will encounter when placing a loved one in a nursing home, they may also experience fear, guilt, or relief as a part of the process. All of these feelings are normal. Learning to deal with them can be difficult. The following excerpts are from an interview with Rick, a Lutheran Pastor who experienced a change in relationship with his mother, as she became increasingly dependent on him.

> When Mom had the stroke about ten years ago, the process of role reversal began almost immediately. It took many years, but it became more and more evident that I was the parent and she was the child. It was interesting, it was a little scary, it was awkward at times. I don't think it was ever awkward for her because of her impairment. The awkwardness was something inside of me.   Rick

When children live in another city or state, the geographic separation may prevent them from seeing the whole picture in terms of their parents' ability to live independently. A decline in the physical or mental health of their elders may go unnoticed for awhile. Emotional distance can create the same situation. Parents or loved ones may want to keep their lives private, hiding their need for assistance. In either case, families are affected by the changes that occur in the relationship with the person needing care.

> I became aware, about 20 years ago, that my folks were not doing well financially. On my recommendation, they picked up stakes and let me move them closer to us. So, that was really the beginning of a long process of change. I moved slowly into that character, first as a counselor, then the decision-maker.   Rick

When the parent begins to look to the child for advice and the child is able to assume the leadership role without anger from the parent, there is a healthy reversal of roles. It is during this natural transition that we begin to accept the aging process. It is an opportunity to come to terms with our fears about our human frailty.

> Quite honestly, well as you know, we hold on to our youth as long as we can, and I became aware of giving up some of the last things of my childhood and of being a son. Accepting it became a part of my aging process. One of the difficult things about dealing with your aging parent is your own aging.   Rick

Most families attempt to avoid the ultimate decision of placement. They may try to keep grandpa and grandma in the community by providing daily assistance. This may be in the form of frequent visits and telephone calls, cooking, cleaning and, finally, hands-on care. The responsibility for this type of support usually falls to the spouse or closest relative. It can be as demanding as caring for a small child.

> After my father died, we brought Mom home. She was with us for seven years. Near the end of that time, I heard my whole family say, "This is getting tough." Mom was increasingly dependent. For many years, I scheduled myself so that I was home at breakfast, lunch and dinner.   Rick

These responsibilities can leave the caregiver exhausted with little time for family, work or self. When all avenues of providing care, at home, have been expended and it is time to make the decision, there may be a feeling of relief.

> When I placed Mom, there was immediate relief. I didn't have to think constantly about her safety or whether she got something to eat.   Rick

Should We Feel Guilty?

Decisions that we make regarding the care of the frail elderly are often complicated by the life's "rules." What our elders taught us about family, the prevailing values of our immediate social group and our religious beliefs all influence these choices. If the choices are not in sync with what has been historically acceptable, the result may be extreme guilt.

> I don't ever remember my mother saying, "Don't put me in a nursing home." I remember my dad saying that. But he died the way we would all like to die, and never had to go to one.   Rick

The decision to place someone in a nursing home brings us face-to-face with our need to be loved or liked by others. Even when we are making a decision that is in the best interests of the individual, we may discover that the decision is unpopular with others who are involved. Parents, family members, and spouse may not agree with what we are about to do. In this instance, we are more apt to feel guilt and uncertainty over the choices we make.

> To the extent that I have felt guilt in the relationship with my mother, and we all do, I don't recognize it as helpful. I understand it as something God can remove. Guilt is regarded as an enemy, particularly in the New Testament. It is something that is alien to us and something that actually becomes a barrier between God and us. In Romans 3, 4, and 5, Paul talks about these barriers that separate us from a full relationship with God. The main thing that Jesus does is remove the barriers: the barrier of sin, the barrier of wrath, the barrier of guilt.   Rick

Often times, what happens in the interaction between adult children and their aging parents is not much different than what happened when the children were younger. The issues we struggle with in relation to our aging parents are the same as those we encountered in our youth. We strive to gain their acceptance, love and approval by doing what they expect of us.

Healthy families exercise the use of positive motivation in decision-making. The children feel a sense of freedom to interact and discuss uncomfortable issues such as how elders will be cared for in the future. These individuals will feel better about the decisions they make on behalf of their parents when the roles are reversed.

Unhealthy families, however, often lack intimate communication, and parents motivate their children with guilt. These children fear punishment and abandonment if they do not measure up. This type of relationship produces dependent and indecisive children who have difficulty parenting their parents when it is necessary to do so.

> My mother is someone who will not face the fact that she may not be able to take care of herself someday. She makes me feel guilty because I won't take her in.
> Susie...age 49

> My grandmother forbade my parents to put her in a nursing home. It put tremendous stress on the family. She lived alone. Then she had a heart attack. While she was in the hospital, the greatest worry of our family was, "What if she survives? None of us were in a position to take care of her, and she had refused placement." Tom...age 41

This type of parenting builds a foundation for false guilt. Guilt is the hook that keeps us from being alone. Its function is to ensure that others will do what we want them to because of our own insecurities that we are not loved. When the younger generation in an unhealthy family is unable or unwilling to do what their elders demand, they have a sense of never being good enough. In unhealthy guilt, we torture ourselves or others. It is a form of abuse, and its purpose is to control.

Is it possible then to have such a thing as healthy guilt? Yes, true guilt originates from God. It is not emotional, but rather a descriptive state, an awareness that we fall short of his expectations. Any other guilt is useless baggage. It depresses us and keeps us from constructive relationships, particularly in regard to parenting our parents when they need us to do so.

Yes all have sinned;
all fall short
of God's glorious ideal,
yet now, God declares us
"not guilty" of offending him
if we trust in Jesus Christ,
who in his kindness
freely takes away our sin.
(Romans 3:23)
Living Bible

Suggestions for Families

The process of caring for our parents and loved ones when they are ill, is an all-consuming and exhausting experience. When placement is necessary, family members may experience the grief of loss and the guilt associated with not being able to provide care.

Be realistic in evaluating what you can and cannot do for your loved one. Set limits related to your time and resources. Do only what you feel you can, and, most of all, ask for help from others.

It is important to remember that, as caregivers, we must also take care of ourselves. By meeting our own needs, maintaining contact with supportive friends and nourishing our lives with periods of rest and relaxation, we will be better able to serve those we love in a healthy, caring way. Many nursing facilities offer support groups for family members. Individual counseling may also be available with the facility social worker, psychologist or chaplain.

If your facility does not have a support group, offer to start one, or contact local agencies such as the Department of Aging, Alzheimer's Association, or nursing-home advocacy groups. (See: Appendix, Children of Aging Parents.)

Additional Resources

Caring for Yourself While Caring for Your Aging Parents, Claire Berman, Henry Holt & Co., New York 1996.

CHAPTER SEVEN

When Loved Ones Become Strangers

*Lord, you know how I long for my
health once more. You hear my
every sigh. My heart beats wildly,
my strength fails, and I am going
blind. My loved ones and friends
stay away, fearing my disease Even
my own family stands at a distance.*

(Psalm 38:9)
Living Bible

Mary Agnes

My mother was a very dignified lady. You wouldn't know it to look at her now. The face of a child smiles back at me from an old woman's body, and hundreds of lines wrinkle the skin around her eyes. I try to remember that face, the way it used to be.

She asks over and over again, "Are you my mother?" trusting me to give her answers to a world she doesn't understand.

I try to be patient. I say, "No, Mother, it's me, Ruth," but she just looks at me and shakes her head. She insists that I call her Mary Agnes. That's what her mama called her when she was a child. Sometimes, she thinks I'm her sister, Rachel. When I tell her Rachel is gone, she gets angry and screams, "You're a liar! You're all liars!" Then she just looks away from me and hums as if I'm not even there. I don't argue anymore. It upsets her so.

My mother was a very beautiful woman. I wish you had known her then. There's a picture on the wall above her bed that looks like me. At night, when she undid her braid, a mass of chestnut hair fell below her waist. Now, it stands out in little silver tufts that she twists with her fingers until the curl comes out.

My mother was a very successful woman. In that picture, she's standing outside her shop on East Avenue. You know that little store on the corner, the one with the striped awning? That was Mary's Tailor Shop until the late '60s. She opened it in 1929 with one month's rent that she had saved from her egg money. She taught me to sew on buttons when I was ten.

My mother was an independent woman. She said you could never rely on anything but your own ambition. She wasn't one to ask people for help. After my father died, we lived in three rooms above the store. It would grieve her to realize just how helpless she is now.

We never had a lot of money, just enough. Mother always said, "Ruth, be grateful for what the Lord gives you, even the hard times." I guess that's why she doesn't complain much now. Troubles never seemed to slow her down. I'm not so flexible. It makes me unhappy to see her like this.

Mother was a very determined woman. When she was thirty-five, she bought the whole building. She was too proud to ask Grandpa for help, even though he was filthy rich. I remember she sewed herself a black wool suit with twenty tiny buttons down the front, just for the occasion. Then she dressed me in my red Sunday jumper and marched right into Mr. Cromwell's office at the bank. She said she didn't want any special consideration because of her social standing or the fact that she was a widow.

My mother was a very trustworthy woman. The bank president loaned her money on just a handshake. She trusts me to take care of her now. She depends on me, but I have betrayed her. The day she walked out of her house without any clothes on, I broke my promise and put her in a nursing home.

My mother was such a lovely woman. I can't believe she slaps and spits when I'm not here. Sometimes, I get so angry with the nurses. I want to say, "This is Mary, not just another old woman that has to be bathed and fed. She's my mother. She was young and vibrant, like all of you. She shouldn't have to wait to have her diapers changed."

My mother was a very particular woman. Every garment that left that tailor shop was perfect. You can see how precise she was by the order of the pictures in her photo album. Every one is labeled and organized by date. I bring it to her when I visit. She mostly likes to talk about the past. The old pictures, the ones when she was a girl on the farm, mean the most to her. She can name every person on the first few pages of the book.

On a good day, we get all the way to the end of the album. She'll point to her grandchildren and repeat their names after me. Sometimes, I think she remembers them, for just a moment. Before her illness, she called them "the delight of her golden years, God's blessings for a job well done." There are four generations of her offspring in that album. The youngest, Mary Agnes, was born last April. Mother loves to hold her when she visits. She calls her Ruth.

My mother was a fun-loving woman. On Saturdays, she would close the shop at noon. We would race across the street to the drug store, sit in the end booth at the soda fountain and order ice cream. In the winter, Mr. Foster would offer us hot chocolate, but Mother said, "It's never too cold for ice cream."

Her favorite was a strawberry sundae. Once, I convinced her to try a cone, but only once. She got chocolate on the end of her nose. We laughed until our sides hurt. Every Saturday, we'd spend an hour there, planning our weekend. Mother said Grandpa never had time for her, only for business, and she wasn't going to raise me like that.

Today was a good day for Mary Agnes. I brought her a strawberry sundae. Before I could unwrap the spoon, she put her face down on the bowl and licked the topping with her tongue. I was impatient when I wiped the whipped cream off her nose. She sat very still for a moment and looked right into my eyes. Then she smiled at me and said, "Didn't we have fun, when I was better?"

My mother was such a dignified lady. I should have bought a cone.

The Isolation Of Aging

Our relentless pursuit of youth has resulted in medical and scientific advances that have improved our health and doubled our life span over the last 100 years. While these advances have enabled us to prolong life, they have also resulted in an increase in diseases related to aging.

The consequences of age-related illnesses have a profound impact on the quality of life for our elders. They may result in the loss of physical abilities such as vision, hearing and movement, or affect judgment and mental capacity. All of these factors separate the elderly from society, restricting their social involvement and ending occupational usefulness. It is this isolation and loss of control that we fear most about growing old.

> I hate to go visit my aunt at the nursing home. Some of
> the people are screaming and yelling. They have no
> physical control. Some are like infants, being fed and
> everything. It's so depressing.   Frank...age 42

There are many changes that we experience in a lifetime of relationships between parents and children, grandparents and grandchildren, husbands and wives, but the greatest changes may occur when a person ages. The deterioration in physical health and mental capacity that precipitates the need for supervised care can greatly alter how individuals relate to each other.

The declines of aging are difficult for all of us to accept, but the loss of physical or intellectual abilities is particularly distressing. When a parent or loved one changes in some way, our relationship with him must change. The balance of give and take that existed to maintain the connection between two individuals is no longer there. One person becomes the caregiver, putting much more into the relationship than the other.

> This is not my father. Anyone will tell you that my dad was a big man: big in stature and big in his heart. I remember the time he flattened a man with one punch because he saw him kicking a dog. I just keep thinking he's going to get better and be like he was. But, you tell me he's not.   Don...age 59

The Changes Of Dementia

The most devastating changes that affect the frail elderly are those that affect the mind. These are caused by a variety of diseases and disorders, such as Alzheimer's, vascular diseases, stroke, Parkinson's and diabetes. Alzheimer's and other related dementias are the most common and affect three out of five nursing-home residents.

Dementia is, perhaps, the most ravaging of diseases affecting elderly in nursing homes. It robs them of relationships, isolates them from society, and financially depletes their assets. It is also the most difficult in regard to providing care. Very few families have the resources necessary to meet the needs of individuals suffering from dementia and to keep them safe. Quite often, their only choice is to place them in a nursing home.

To have a dementia diagnosis, a person must exhibited a loss of abilities in at least two areas of complex behavior, such as language, memory, visual and spatial abilities, or judgment. Over time, the symptoms get worse until the individual requires total care.

Because dementia is a disease with regressing behaviors, individuals may in the later stages appear childlike and lose their inhibitions. Where they previously maintained a very proper facade in public, they may now exhibit actions that are socially inappropriate and embarrassing to those around them. Quite often, dementia patients are very outspoken. They may be rude and critical of others.

> I recall a woman who was in the early stages of dementia. She said whatever was on her mind at the time without regard to the feelings of others. One day, a visitor said, good morning to her, and she told the woman, "You are entirely too fat to wear a dress with flowers on it!"   Ann...Social Worker

Gradually, dementia patients lose the ability to comprehend language and express thought. Their world is one of frustration and change. The people they loved and the places they lived are no longer familiar to them, yet their emotional and physical needs do not stop with the progression of the disease. The behaviors they exhibit are an expression of these needs. Like all of us, they react to discomfort, hunger, thirst, fear or loneliness. For example, the person with dementia may wander because he is looking for something familiar, or cry out in response to pain.

Some residents with dementia are extremely noisy. They pound repetitively on objects near them or scream obscenities. Others exhibit physical and/or sexual aggression including hitting, grabbing or fondling of caregivers. Family and friends find these behaviors most distressing. It is upsetting to see a grown person act in a childlike manner, particularly when the individual was very different in the past.

> My mother was kind and loving, a very sweet-tempered woman. She would just do anything for anyone. I couldn't imagine her biting or hitting or pulling someone's hair.   Mary...age 50

Accepting The Change

We want our loved ones to be the way we remember them. Our relationship is based on those past experiences. To watch them decline, to see them change, causes us to grieve. For some families, the pain is unbearable, and they stay away.

> I don't visit my husband much anymore because he doesn't know me.   Katherine...age 75

For many years, nursing homes kept residents with dementia tied up and over-medicated. These practices, intended to control behavior, actually intensified the symptoms of dementia. In addition, being restrained and inactive for long periods of time led to further health problems, such as bedsores, pneumonia and other infections. These methods of caring for the aged became the driving force behind nursing-home reform of the 1980s.

Today, because of state and federal regulations, the use of restraints, in nursing homes, whether physical or chemical, is prohibited. Our understanding of dementia helps us to be more realistic about the changing abilities and needs of these individuals. The focus is on treating residents with dignity and respect by meeting their physical and emotional needs. To accomplish this is an awesome task that requires a commitment from all of us.

Sometimes it's hard to remember the person behind the disease, to know the individual as he or she used to be. As family members and caregivers, we must remember that the person with dementia is a person with a past, a person with passions and dreams, someone like ourselves. When we visit our loved ones and care for them, we minister to them in their frailty. In this way we honor God and give thanks for their life. One daughter expressed this in a beautiful thank-you letter written to the staff who cared for her mother.

> I have often asked myself, "Why did my mother have to suffer so?" But I see now that God makes everything beautiful. Maybe He prolonged her life so we could learn more about love...family...friends...choices. You have taught me much about these things. Even when she was difficult, you loved her and cared for her. God bless all of you, and thank you from the bottom of my heart. Angela...age 57

I have created you
and cared for you
since you were born.
I will be your God
though all your lifetime, yes,
even when your hair
is white with age.

(Isaiah 46:3-4)
Living Bible

Suggestions for Families

Meeting the needs of persons with dementia and providing for their safe care is a task that requires 24-hour supervision and interventions. When elderly family members need placement for their own safety and well being, you can continue to be involved.

Don't stay away because others have taken over the task of caring for your loved one. Your presence is very important, even if your parent forgets who you are or seems to be unaware that you are visiting.

Learn to accept your parent or loved one as he is now. Listen when he talks. Join him in discussions of the past. Embrace the good moments. Share memories. Give hugs and lots of reassurance.

Your presence can be a help to everyone. Who knows your father better than you do? Help to communicate his needs, his wishes, his likes and dislikes to the people who take care of him.

Additional Resources

Alzheimer's, A Caregiver's Sourcebook, Howard Gruetzner, John Wiley & Sons Inc., New York, 1992.

The Validation Breakthrough: Simple Techniques for Communicating With People With Alzheimer's-Type Dementia, Naomi Feil, Health Professions Press, 1994.

The 36 Hour Day: A Family Guide to Caring for Persons With Alzheimer's Disease, Related Dementing Illnesses, and Memory Loss in Later Life, Nancy L. Mace, Peter V. Rabins, John Hopkins University Press, 1991.

My Journey into Alzheimer's Disease, Robert Davis, Tyndale House, 1984.

CHAPTER EIGHT

The Care
Of Strangers

I was hungry and you fed me,
thirsty and you gave me a drink;
I was a stranger and you received
me into your homes, naked and you
clothed me; I was sick and you took
care of me, in prison and you visited
me...I tell you, whenever you did
this for one of the least important of
these brothers of mine, you did it
for me!

(Matthew 25:35-36, 40)
Good News Bible

Marcella

Today was pretty much like any other day. Marcella opened her eyes a few moments before 5:30, just as she had done for nearly a century. Then she pushed the covers to the side of her bed, thinking it was time to get up for work.

"Wait until I can help you," called a voice from the dimly lit hallway.

Marcella dangled her bony legs over the edge of the mattress. "I don't need any help. I've got to get ready for school."

A middle-aged woman bustled into the room pushing a walker up to Marcella's bedside. "Not today, Honey. That was a long time ago. You're not a teacher any more. You live in a nursing home now."

"I forgot, again. I think you tell me that every day, Arlene." Marcella winced, as she pushed herself off the bed and put weight onto her aching feet.

"Don't be in a big hurry, you'll fall. I just wish you'd stay in bed once. Then I could get some of these other people taken care of. You're in such a rush to get up."

"Did I ever tell you that my mother always said we didn't needed a rooster after I was born?"

"A hundred times, dear. Sit here on the toilet and wash up." Arlene dampened a wash cloth with cold water and laid a towel on the sink. "Put the light on when you're done."

"What day is it?"

"Thursday, August 5th." Arlene moved toward the door.

"What year?"

"1995." She called over her shoulder. "Don't forget to put your call light on."

"It's my birthday," Marcella said to an empty room.

A half-hour later, Arlene returned. Marcella rose stiffly from sitting on the commode, shuffled back to her bed and sat on the edge while she dressed. Her slip strap was broken.

"Do you have a safety pin?"

"No, I don't, Honey. You'll have to let it hang." Arlene picked a faded pink housedress from the closet and slipped it over Marcella's head.

"Your clothes are a wreck," she said, trying to close the front of the dress with two buttons instead of four. "Why don't those boys of yours bring you some new things? I know the nurse has asked them many times."

Marcella pulled at the front of her dress to cover the gap. "They don't come to visit me."

"I can't find any matching socks, Dear, so we'll have to put these stockings on. Do you have garters?"

"I don't think so."

Arlene rolled one nylon down to a small circle and slipped it over Marcella's left foot. Then she pulled it up over her leg and twisted the top into a tight knot that rested just above her kneecap. After repeating this with the other stocking, she helped Marcella put on her slippers and assisted her to a standing position.

"You can sit out there in the dining room and wait for breakfast. It will be ready in about an hour."

Marcella pushed her walker ahead of her, shoulders bent, head down, sliding her feet along so the slippers wouldn't flop when she moved. Her right stocking came undone. She stopped to twist it into another knot, leaned too far forward and lost her balance against a chair. A nurse helped her to a seated position and asked how she was.

"I'm just fine. Did you know it's my birthday?"

"Well, happy birthday, Honey. I wish I had time to visit."

After breakfast, a volunteer brought Marcella a red silk rose with a pink ribbon tied to it and a small package wrapped in white tissue paper. The card said, "Birthday Wishes from the Glenfield Lioness Club."

Marcella pulled off the curly ribbon and opened the gift. Inside the package were two pairs of white ankle socks and a sample bottle of dry skin lotion.

"Happy Birthday, Marcella," the volunteer said. "When the mail comes, I'll bring you your cards. And don't forget, we celebrate birthdays on the third Thursday of the month."

"Thank you."

At noon, there was a small tin-foil pan on the corner of her lunch tray. In it was a frosted cake covered with plastic wrap. A waitress, from the kitchen, peeled the bakery sticker off the wrapping and shouted, "Hey, it's Marcella's birthday today!" and everyone started singing.

"Happy birthday to you. Happy birthday to you. Happy birthday, Marcella...."

She smiled and thanked them for remembering. The smell of meat loaf and baked potatoes reminded Marcella of her sixteenth birthday. It was on a Sunday. Mother had invited Aunt Mary, Uncle George and her cousin Grace for dinner. Papa bought her a garnet ring with six beautiful stones that were set to look like a flower. When her first grandchild was born, Marcella gave the ring to her daughter-in-law.

After lunch, Marcella waited in the front lobby for her guests. Visitors came and went, but none of them sat next to her. Bertha's daughter, Nancy, asked about the rose. Marcella told her it was her ninety-fifth birthday and showed her the white socks. Nancy gave her a hug and a kiss.

By five o'clock, Marcella knew there would be no mail. The lobby was empty, and the nurse hadn't called her to answer the phone. When dinner was over, she shuffled back to her room, took off the stockings that kept falling down and put on her nightgown. Tomorrow, she would wear the socks.

The Eldercare Dilemma

We live in an era of social causes. Movie stars raise money to feed hungry children in Africa. The rich and famous endorse efforts to find a cure for terminal diseases. Minority groups march for their right to equal or privileged treatment. Veterans' organizations demand recognition and restitution for service to their country. Anti-abortionists go to jail for the rights of the unborn. But the fastest growing segment of the population, the frail elderly, lacks the support necessary to protect them from being victimized and abused by those who should be sensitive to their needs.

Over the last century, increasing longevity has brought about new problems for our society. We are beginning to face the difficulties of caring for large numbers of individuals who no longer make a contribution but require investments of time, energy and money to maintain their lives. As growing numbers of elders move into their eighties and nineties, there is a rising demand for organizations that offer supportive services. At the same time, there is a decline in the numbers of younger people available to provide those services.

In a perfect world, the aged and infirm should continue to live among family and friends who love them unconditionally and meet their every need, but the reality is far from perfect. From the poor houses of the 1700s to present day nursing facilities, America's solution to eldercare has focused on institutionalization.

To end our lives in a nursing home is a destiny most of us fear, yet it is a choice we make for millions of our loved ones, because we cannot or will not make the sacrifices necessary to care for them.

> Institutionalization of the elderly in this country amounts to benign avoidance. We put them in a facility so that others can take care of them. There is a benefit to this. It takes the stress off and relieves us of our responsibilities. We look to others who are kind to take over the job that we are unwilling to do.
> Rick...geriatric psychiatrist

Is it realistic to think we can solve the problems of eldercare by continuing to build bigger and better facilities? This seems to be our goal, and corporate America is cashing in on the financial benefits. Providing medical care to the growing numbers of frail elderly is a profitable business that is plagued with multiple problems.

Paying strangers to do what we cannot or will not do ourselves, has its price. The high cost of care, fraudulent business practices, the hiring of unskilled and unfit caregivers, reports of abuse and neglect are but a few of the problems that trouble the nursing-home industry. The shortcomings of the system are only symptoms of a larger problem.

"Elder abuse is America's dirty secret." [1] It includes financial exploitation, physical, mental and sexual abuse and neglect. Abuse occurs in communities, in homes, in hospitals and in institutions and is a growing concern among professionals. "According to a 1990 congressional report, about one out of every twenty older Americans may be a victim of elder abuse every year." [2] "Nearly all cases of elder abuse involve greed." [3] Whether it is a family member who stands to gain financially from the assets of an individual, a nurse's aide who pockets a resident's valuables or a corporation that maintains its profit line by paying low wages to caregivers, money is the major factor in victimization.

The Need For Social Advocacy

The biggest contributing factor is personal apathy. Support for social reform in regard to care of the aging is sadly lacking. This is not surprising in view of our fears about aging and death. To be old in our society is to have no future and, therefore, no further value. In an effort to avoid anything that reminds of this fact, we close our minds to the problems of growing old. It is easier for us to support those social issues that we see as hopeful, or those over which we have some control, such as saving baby whales.

For the one and one-half million Americans over the age of sixty-five who live in institutions, the question of social advocacy is a critical one. The physical and mental vulnerability of this group of individuals makes them particularly prone to victimization.

Social reform has taken the path of government regulations to control the long-term care industry. In the past decade, federal and state regulations have had a positive impact on raising the standards for care in institutions.

The law has been effective for those institutions, both private and for profit, which are dedicated to providing quality care. But for the hundreds of nursing facilities where care is substandard, government regulation is cumbersome and, in many cases, ineffective.

What goes on inside a nursing home is really of little concern to most individuals. As long as we don't have to think about abuse and neglect of the elderly, we can deny that it exists. From time to time, the media jolts us from our passivity with horror stories about institutional care: residents who have been beaten or raped, who have been allowed to lie in their own excrement, who die because they do not receive the most basic of medical and personal care.

More common in nursing homes, is the day-to-day, collective neglect and apathy that is a result of overworked, underpaid care-giving staff.

> What do I think of living in a nursing home? It stinks. You ask them to take you to the bathroom, and they tell you to wait. Then, when they put you on the toilet, they tell you to hurry up.   Gordon...age 86

> A nurse's aide gave me a bed bath. Then she dipped my comb in the dirty bath water and combed my hair. Sometimes, she'd do that with my toothbrush. Aaron...age 77

Many times the abuse is unintentional. It may be a scolding tone of voice, an attitude of impatience, a delay in performing needed cares. Over time, when you have an accumulation of these "little" abuses, the effect can be the same as a violent act. There is a loss of dignity, a sense of helplessness when residents are dependent on caregivers for everything and those caregivers are insensitive to their feelings or needs.

The role of caregiver to the elderly is the most physically and emotionally demanding job within the nursing-home setting. Today's nursing-home residents are the most critically ill or difficult to manage of the elderly population. Many have behavior problems that present a physical threat to those who provide hands-on care. It is not surprising that we delegate these tasks to others.

We rely on these strangers to perform the most intimate of tasks for our loved ones: bathing, feeding, clothing and diapering. In addition, we expect them to provide comfort, spend quality time, and solve their problems. It would seem that we believe money is a substitute for love and responsibility, and that we can pay organizations and caregivers to be the family that we are not.

> I pay $5,000 a month for you to take care of my mother. I don't have time to visit her every day. Please don't have her call me when she wants to go home. Henry...age 54

Thousands of men and women devote their lives to the compassionate care of the elderly, and they do it for the lowest wages and the least recognition of any profession. For them, it is not a job, but a calling. For all of us, it is an example.

> I am often asked, "How can you stand working in a nursing home?" I try to explain to people that we are a community, just like any other. There is friendship and conflict, hope and despair, laughter and tears. It is part

of life. It's what you make of it. Despite the fact that we begin as strangers, for most of us, there is a sense of family.   Lynn...social worker

Residents recognize the dedication and sensitivity of caregivers who are committed to their work. Many had praise for those who took care of them.

> None of us wants to be here. We'd all rather be someplace else. There are a lot of things I like, and there's a lot of good staff. People who give you a hug, who stop to talk, who just take time to listen. James...age 44

> When I first came here, I hated it because I was separated from my family, and I didn't want to leave my home. Now, I've made countless friends, especially with the workers. I like it when the girls kiss me good night. Mae...age 84

> People used to talk about nursing homes. I had a cousin who went to visit a friend in one, and that woman just hated being there. I can't think of a single reason why anyone would hate it. The workers do such nice things for us. Besides, if my mother knew I had a man putting me to bed every night, she'd turn over in her grave. Alice...age 86

Our Personal Responsibility

The responsibility for compassionate care of the elderly belongs to all of us. We can blame the government or corporations for failures in the system, but it is personal involvement that will bring results. We can pay for services, but we cannot buy values or legislate caring. These have to be demonstrated. The greatest single need in nursing homes is companionship. In some facilities, less than half of the residents have regular visitors.

> These little grandmas are crying for their mothers. They
> need someone to love them. It's so sad when no one
> visits them.   Beth...nursing assistant

Family and friends who come to visit provide a valuable contribution to the well being of residents and emotional support to the staff. Author, Timothy Diamond, observed this in his book, *Making Gray Gold*. "To watch these wives and daughters, nieces and husbands circulate through the halls with their particular greeting for particular people, remembering a birthday, nicknames, a specific problems with sickness was to see them create an integral part of the social fabric of these homes." [4]

Visitors are the eyes and ears of the community. Nursing-home advocacy groups promote visitation because residents who have guests get better care. Family members, friends, and volunteers can make a difference. To be present in nursing facilities on a regular basis is to show that someone cares about what happens inside our society's institutions. It makes everyone accountable. It brings about change.

Some families are there every day, feeding their loved ones, helping with care, asking questions, watching out for those who have no one else. It's about personal and social responsibility to others. This is what Christ is speaking of in Matthew 25. He talks about "hands-on" involvement that requires a commitment of our time. To care for the elderly, "the least of these," is to care for Him.

One thing families don't realize is that they have to be advocates for everything: diet, care, medications, clothing, every aspect of the nursing home. At first, it was me against them. I was really afraid to talk to these people because they were staff. But then, gradually, we became friends, and we were working together: nurses, nursing assistants, social workers, even the cleaning help. It became a friendly place.   Norma...age 62

Suggestions for Families

There is no place like home, and no one will ever care for our loved ones the way we would like to care for them. You have a right to be involved. Some family members feel it is enough to visit on a regular basis. Others wish to continue their hands-on responsibilities, even after placement. You may want to fix your mother's hair, help to feed her, assist in dressing, or even bathing. Talk to your facility, and make your wishes known.

Be supportive of your parent's caregivers. Give praise and encouragement to staff who are doing a good job. Volunteer your time to show that you care. Communicate with staff about your parent, what is important to you and your expectations for how his or her needs will be met.

The most significant thing for families to remember is that residents in nursing homes who have frequent visitors, get better care. Visitors are the eyes and ears of the community. Their presence helps to make caregivers accountable for what goes on inside a facility. If you have reservations about the care your family member is receiving, or the way a facility deals with other residents, there are agencies that can help you work for a better outcome. (See Appendix: National Association of State Units on Aging and National Citizens' Coalition for Nursing-home Reform)

Additional Resources

The Long-Term Care Family Manual, MaryLou Hughes, Professional Printing & Publishing, 1991.

Nursing Homes: Getting Good Care There, Sarah Greene Burger, Virginia Fraser, Sara Hunt, Barbara Frank, American Source Books, 1996.

CHAPTER NINE

The Shadow Of Death

Yea, though I walk through
the valley of the shadow
of death, I will fear no evil:
for thou art with me; thy rod and
thy staff they comfort me.

(Psalm 23:4)
King James

Markus

The last time I saw Markus, it was snowing. We sat together and watched big white flakes melt against the window of the visiting room and run down in little rivers to the sill.

"They remind me of tears," he said.

I looked at the man who was so like my grandfather, gentle and soft-spoken. He sat with his elbows resting on the arms of his wheelchair, hands clasped in front of him as he stared out the window.

I had been counseling Markus for over four weeks, and I wasn't any closer to knowing what kept him awake at night. The caregivers told me they would get him to bed about nine and by ten he was back in his wheelchair, parked by the desk, asking for a drink of ice water or cough medicine. Through the night, he would read his newspaper or nap in a chair by the television, refusing to lie down again until he saw the sun come up.

Each day Markus appeared more tired, the circles darkening around his large brown eyes. Bruises covered his arms, and he wheezed as he forced air in and out of his lungs.

"They tell me I'm going to die, Dr. Langmade. Do you think it's true?" His voice broke with a spasm of coughing.

I waited for him to catch his breath, giving myself time to consider how I would answer. But he continued as if he hadn't asked the question at all.

"Of course, we're all going to die someday, some of us sooner than others." He paused and shook his head from side to side. "Not me. I'm going to beat this thing. I just got to get rid of this cough and get some rest. I can't seem to rest."

I leaned back in my chair and let him talk.

"It's just a matter of time," Markus continued. "Lots of people recover from cancer. I was reading the other day about some new cure they're working on. Even my daughter told me she thought I looked better since I came to the nursing home. I told her, 'Of course I do. I'm working hard in physical therapy.' You gotta follow the rules and have a good outlook, if you want to get well."

The coughing started again. Markus pulled a yellow nebulizer from his pocket, shook it several times, sprayed it into his mouth, and inhaled. His breath whistled as he strained to blow it out again.

"You know, Doc, I really appreciate you stopping to see me every day. It means a lot, like we're getting to be good friends or something."

"I consider you a friend, Markus. In fact, you remind me of my grandfather."

"Is that a fact?" He looked at me, and a smile brightened his face. For a moment the tiredness seemed to disappear. "Why, I'd be right proud to call a fine man like yourself 'grandson', Doc. Do you think when I get out of here we could still be friends? Maybe we could have lunch together or something, once in a while. I never did have much time for friends. It's one of the things I regret about my life, not taking time to smell the roses as they say." He leaned forward in his chair, lifting his shoulders to get more air.

"I'd like that, Markus."

The coughing started again. Markus picked a cough drop from a bag that was beside him in the chair and offered me one. I declined. His hands shook as he unwrapped the twisted paper ends and popped one into his mouth.

"Yeah," he continued, shifting the cough drop to his cheek, "I guess we all have things we wish we'd done different. Like my wife, Sadie. I didn't do right by her. Oh, she always told me she was happy. I guess that's because I made a good living, but I was always working, always worried about money."

He took a deep breath and, as he exhaled, the smell of Mentholyptus filled the room. "I worked seven days a week. Never did go to church much, even though Sadie asked me to. She took care of that for the children. I figured God wants a man to provide for his family. I never was baptized neither. Pa said he didn't have the time to get it done. Day comes when you know you should have done different."

"It's not too late, Markus. You could still be baptized."

He looked at me. "Doc, I really appreciate you talking to me about God and that forgiveness stuff. Nobody's ever explained it to me that way, about it being a gift and all. I still don't see how that's possible. I never got nothing without working for it."

He lowered his head into the palms of his hands and shut his eyes. There was a long silence, and I wondered if he had fallen asleep. I listened for his breathing.

His voice was barely a whisper now. "You remember the other day when you asked me if I wanted to talk about the thing that's got me worried?"

"I remember."

"Well, I gave it some thought, Doc. You're the best friend a man ever had and I trust you, but I just can't do it. I can't tell you. Things would never be the same between us."

He looked up again, blinking tears from his eyes. "I'm getting pretty tired. The next time I see you, I want to ask you some more questions about that King David. You know, the one that was God's favorite. Did he really kill somebody and still go to heaven?"

"It's a fact, Markus. There's nothing you could do that God won't forgive."

"That's pretty hard to believe." He turned his chair and headed back to his room. "I gotta lay down now, Doc. If I could just rest awhile, maybe I could feel better. I just can't seem to shut my eyes at night."

∾

The Final Separation

It is death's shadow that distorts our view of aging and causes us to be reminded of our frailty as human beings, and death is what we fear most about nursing homes. Facing the death of our parents or loved ones brings about the necessity to wrestle with the core issues of our own humanity and, ultimately, our relationship to God. Death represents a final separation from all that is known and safe. Furthermore, to die in a nursing home means that we have been uprooted from our families and placed with strangers who will care for us in our final hours of life.

Over the past century, our society has distanced itself from death. Because of changes in medical technology, care of the sick and elderly, once a family responsibility, has been shifted to the professional community. As a result, we have seen the development of multi-million dollar businesses, such as hospitals and nursing homes, that deal with death and dying. By 1984, seventy-one percent of deaths in the United States occurred in institutions. [1]

Author Joseph Bayly writes, "In this generation death moved out of the home to the hospital; doctors and nurses replaced the family, and a dying father became a terminal patient. The ordinary, age-old fear of death gained an added dimension; the anticipation of being alone in life's closing hour, isolated from those with whom the other hours and years and decades of life were shared." [2]

Our apprehension about death is as old as the history of mankind. It stems from the trauma of being alienated from God in the Garden of Eden, and has resulted in our inherent avoidance of anything that reminds us of that estrangement. We fear death, and we fear the isolation of dying alone. Both represent a final separation from all that is familiar and safe and, ultimately, a separation from God.

The Denial Of Death

Thus, we stand at a distance from death, not wanting to view the process or participate in the care of the dying. In their book, *When A Friend Is Dying*, authors Edward Dobihal and Charles Stewart explain that we look to hospitals and institutions to provide this service of terminal care, and we expect them to produce medical miracles that will delay death even longer. "They (institutions) do often extend life and that is very good. Sometimes they extend dying and that can be very bad. They do not eliminate death and that is very factual." [3]

Within the nursing-home environment where caring for the dying is a specialty, we continue to exhibit a denial of death. Federal regulations governing nursing homes require that we "improve the quality of life" for residents and keep them at their highest functioning level. We insist on medical interventions that delay the natural dying process as long as possible, and we feed residents when they no longer want to eat.

Caregivers must deny their grief to protect other residents and to perform their duties in a professional manner. They minister to the terminal patient and then move on to the next individual without allowing themselves to show their emotion or share the experience of the loss. Even our choice of vocabulary expresses this denial.

> They use terms such as "passed away" and "expired" in the long-term care setting. License plates expire! Nobody ever says the word "dead." It's like we can't admit it happens here.   Chari...nurse

In *Making Grey Gold*, a book about long-term care, author, Timothy Diamond, observes, "Deaths occurred as silenced, hushed events, as though they were failures in this secular medical system. Yet, another lesson for residents to learn was that praying and mourning for the deceased were done primarily alone." [4]

> I used to be skittish about death. Now it doesn't bother me as much. They don't say anything when someone goes, but I notice things like who's missing at the breakfast table.   Bea...86

For family members and friends there is often the struggle of not wanting to see their loved ones suffer, yet not wanting them to leave. They may argue at the deathbed among themselves about the individual's right to die and even pressure the resident to accept hospitalization or more treatment. There comes a time when we must release parents or loved ones from the responsibilities of living, a time when we can no longer make demands upon them.

> I remember one woman who could not cope with her mother's refusal of life-support measures. She sat by her bedside and screamed at her, "Don't leave me, Mama." Karen...nursing assistant.

At the other extreme are families who want to hasten the process of dying. They are grieved by their witness to suffering and assume that it is their right to end it. One nurse recalled an incident when a daughter asked that her father be given an extra dose of morphine because she knew it would suppress his respiration and heart rate more quickly.

> Please tell families not to ask professionals to hasten the death of their relatives. It places a terrible burden on us emotionally, professionally, and morally.   Shelly...nurse

Death As A Door

Many elderly nursing-home residents are not afraid to die. They long for death to end their suffering and loneliness. For them, the nursing home is a place of waiting.

> I'm ready to die. I've lived too many years and I want to just shut my eyes and never wake up.   Millie...102

Our distance from God creates a void that we spend a lifetime trying to fill. Like Markus, we sense that our sin has forever separated us from God's presence and know in our hearts that this is the cause of our loneliness and pain. We immerse ourselves in the things of life so that we don't have to deal with thinking about how fragile life is. The relentless pursuit of success, ownership of more things, seeking love in the wrong places, obsessions with health and fitness are all efforts to prevent, or at least delay, the day when we must stand at death's door and face eternity.

Death is the one thing we can't control, and we like to be in control. This fact forces us to make a choice. We can rely on the things we are able to see, feel and touch for satisfaction, things that will ultimately fail us. Or, day by day, we can transfer that trust to God who is eternal and will never fail us; a God who humbled Himself and became a man, who taught us how to die, who saves us from our sins, who offers us eternal life.

As we make the transition to faith, we will recognize the futility of material things. Instead of searching for perfection, we will seek a relationship with the One who is truly perfect. Instead of clinging to life and family and things, we will truly be free to love each other. Like residents who must let go of their possessions to move to the nursing home, we must all let go of life to move on to eternity. It is the ultimate paradox – to die that we might live. Jesus said, "I am the resurrection and the life. Whoever believes in me will live, even though he dies; and whoever lives and believes in me will never die." (John 11: 25, 26 – Good News Bible)

The author of the twenty-third Psalm knew this truth. Even though he readily admitted his fear of walking through the valley, he understood that his future was with the Shepherd and that he would not be alone in the process.

Surely goodness and mercy
shall follow me
all the days of my life:
and I will dwell in the house
of the Lord forever.
(Psalm 23:6)
King James

Suggestions for Families

Death in an institution can be lonely and impersonal. When a loved one is facing the end of his or her life, family and friends become more important than ever before. This is a time to share feelings, to resolve issues, to review a lifetime of experiences and to talk in the most intimate of ways.

Our fear of death can limit our ability to deal openly with someone who is dying. If we avoid death and stay away, we increase our anxiety. Through knowledge and involvement we can come to terms with our own beliefs about life and death. This is necessary before we can be of help to others.

There is no right or wrong way to deal with the dying person. Let him be your guide. Encourage conversation. Listen when your loved one wants to talk. Answer his questions honestly. Read his favorite Bible passages. Reassure him and yourself, with hope of eternal life.

Allow the individual to have as many choices as possible. Ask what his wishes are regarding medical procedures, pain control, and funeral arrangements. What will make him comfortable? Who does he want to visit with?

We have included some excellent references to help you understand how death happens and how you can minister to the dying person. For additional information, see Visiting Nurse Association and American Hospice Foundation (Appendix).

Additional Resources

Final Gifts: Understanding the Special Awareness, Needs, and Communications of the Dying, Maggie Callanan, Patricia Kelley, Bantam Books, 1997.

When a Friend Is Dying, Edward F. Dobihal, Abingdon Press, 1984.

My Journey Into Alzheimer's Disease, Robert Davis, Tyndale House, 1984.

Suggested Bible readings:
    Psalm 23
    John 11: 21-17 and 14: 1-6
    Romans 8: 35-39
    1 John 5: 10-13

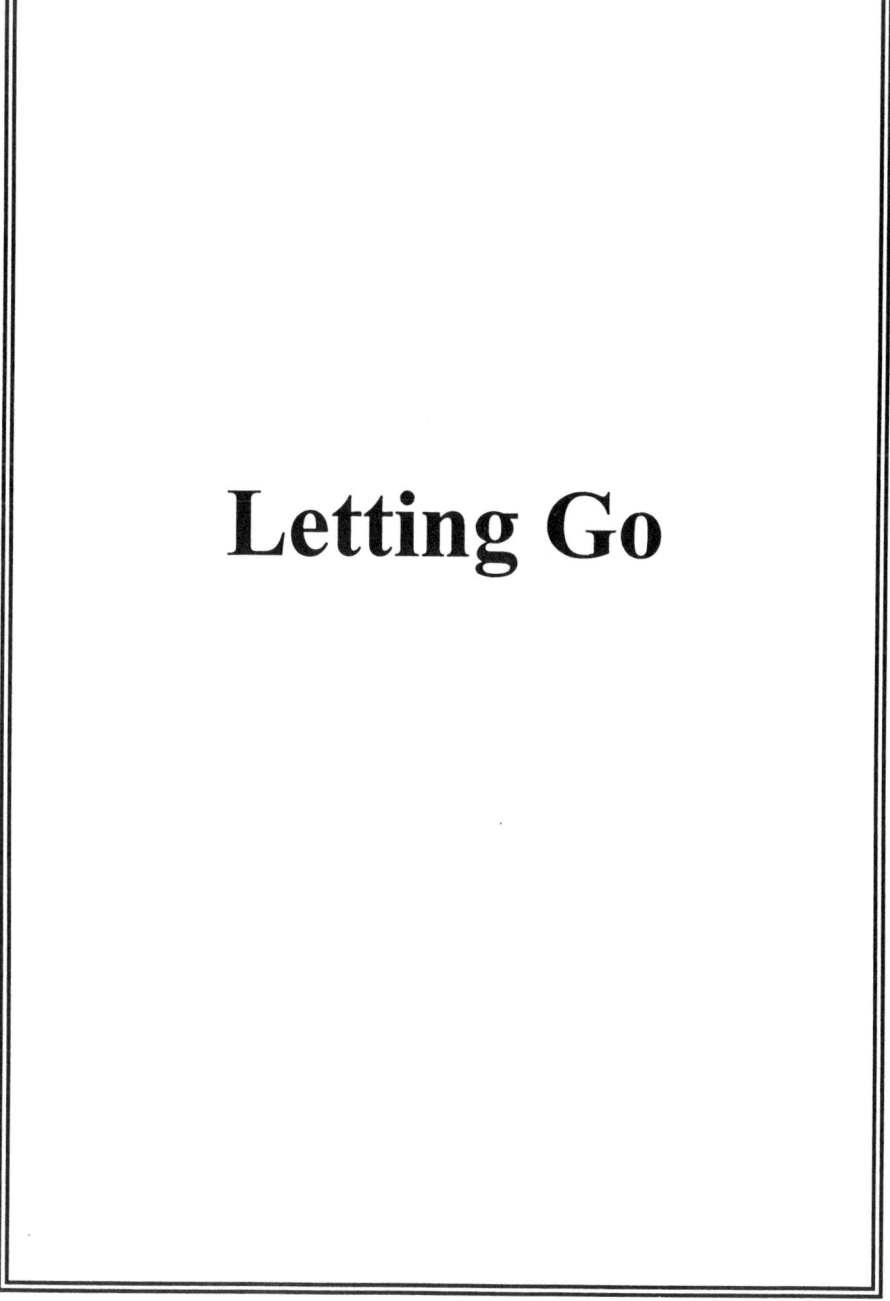

Letting Go

*How weary we grow of our present
bodies. That is why we look
forward eagerly to the day when we
shall have heavenly bodies which
we shall put on like new clothes.
And we are not afraid, but are quite
content to die, for then we will be
at home with the Lord.*

(2 Corinthians 5: 2,8)
Living Bible

Gertrude

I remember the morning that Gertrude decided to die. She informed her aide, Dora, that she would certainly not be taking breakfast or getting out of bed. The distraught young woman hurried down the corridor and burst into my office without knocking.

"Linda, Mrs. Santi is being difficult again," Dora complained. "She refuses to get up or eat her breakfast. Says she's ready for the cemetery and wants to see you."

"Tell her I'll be there as soon as I can. I have a few things to do."

"She says to hurry. She wants to make sure she gets a chance to say good-bye."

"Thank you, Dora."

I took in a deep breath, mentally counting to ten. Could I have just one morning that didn't start with Gertrude's problems? I wondered about the urgency in Dora's request, but dismissed it. Gertrude certainly wasn't dying yesterday, when I saw her at breakfast.

"I ordered farina, not oatmeal," she had shouted, shaking a crooked finger at me. "And there isn't enough jelly for my toast."

"I'll be happy to get what you want from the kitchen, Gertrude."

"It's too late now," she said, pulling off her bib and throwing it on her tray. "You should have thought of that sooner."

"Why don't you try eating in the dining room, Gertrude? You could choose what you want and get it right away."

"It's too noisy, and I don't want to eat with all those old people," she grumbled.

Today, Gertrude would have to wait. I had phone calls to make and other residents to see. Besides, every day was a crisis for Gertrude. She had been with us for only two of her ninety-three years and in that time had caused more problems than all of our other residents combined.

Nearly every morning, Gertrude would have the entire staff in an uproar and the nursing assistants in tears. "The girls," as she called them, were always disrespectful. The food wasn't fit to eat. Her roommate was an "old biddy" and her tummy always hurt.

After breakfast, Gertrude would fuss and fume about the particulars of her dressing. Things had to be just so. She insisted that bright circles of pink rouge be painted on her cheekbones, and Cherry Crimson was the only shade of lipstick she would ever consider wearing. A tiny bow had to be pinned to the very top of her silver curls, and brooches belonged in the center front of her sweatshirt.

Once she was dressed, she was ready to see the social worker. Sometimes Gertrude just wanted to talk about her indigestion or her "arthur-itis," as she called it. But, generally, it was a crisis that had her in tears.

"I just can't stand it here anymore, Linda. Everyone's so mean to me." Her Cherry Crimson lips pursed into a frown. "That woman across the hall is a thief. She stole the box of candy I got for my birthday."

"Gertrude, you said you didn't like that candy. I saw you give it to her."

"Well, I shouldn't have, and I want it back!"

My own feelings about Gertrude alternated between compassion and impatience. She was a curious mixture of saint and sinner. On the one hand, she faithfully attended all of the religious services in our facility, regardless of denomination and on the other, she liked to stir things up. I felt sorry for her because she was lonely, but I found it easy to judge her behaviors, especially when Gertrude's son told me about her years of anger and control.

After finishing some phone calls and paperwork, I headed toward Gertrude's room. Mary, her nurse, met me outside the door. Removing her stethoscope, she spoke in whispered tones.

"Mrs. Santi is dying. Her skin is mottled, her hands are cold, blood pressure is low. She asked me to call her son."

I entered her room. Gertrude lay quietly in bed, her silver curls and translucent skin pale against the white sheets and coverlet. In her hands she grasped a blue rosary. For the first time, I noticed her frailty.

"Good morning, Gertrude. I heard you wanted to see me."

"Oh, Linda, I'm so glad you came." Her eyes were glazed and didn't seem to focus.

"I told Mary I don't want nothin' done. And I told Cora not to fuss over me, making me wear all that rouge and stuff. Just told her to wash me up so I don't stink when people come to visit. I don't need no lipstick or anything where I'm going." She took a deep breath. "I just wanted to thank all you girls for being so nice to me. And...and I wanted to tell you I love you."

I stroked her forehead. "I love you, Gertrude. Are you in pain?"

"No, I'm just fine."

"God loves you, too," I whispered.

"Oh, I know that!" she snapped. "And I know where I'm going. Every day of my life, when I went to bed, I squeezed my eyes shut and said my 'God Blesses' for everyone, and for all of you girls too." With a wave of her hand, she dismissed me, saying there were others she wanted to see.

Throughout the day and into evening, word passed among the employees. One by one, they quietly filed into Gertrude's room, saying their private good-byes. Her family came and went.

By nine o'clock she was gone. Gertrude, the most difficult individual I had ever met...a sinner, a believer, a child of God. She lived and died with certainty. There were no apologies or regrets, simply grace.

Accepting Death

Residents who are accepting of death often know when it is time to die. It is quite common for elderly people to talk about praying for death as a release from their suffering. This can be physical suffering, the loss of family and friends, or both. Many feel that they have lived long enough. Some are frustrated that death does not come when they hope for it.

Sometimes, individuals are able to will death for themselves. They may shove people away, become distant, refuse to talk and even stop eating. This behavior is frequently observed with dementia patients who will turn away when fed or spit food from their mouths. The decision to eat or not to eat is the last area of control that residents are able to exercise over their lives.

For families this is a difficult time. Saying good-bye to those we love is one of life's most painful experiences. In recent generations, our knowledge of death is usually limited to visiting a funeral home when someone we know has passed away. The rest of the time we act as if death doesn't exist. As a result, we do not spend adequate time grieving the losses of our past. The grief we feel when our parents or loved ones die is a culmination of all the losses we experience over a lifetime. It is this, combined with the fear of our own death, that makes the experience hurt so much.

Institutional walls provide a barrier to the less attractive side of life. When death occurs in a nursing home, it is easy to stay away. We don't have to witness the end when others are paid to provide this service. By avoiding death, we deceive ourselves. We think, "Maybe it won't happen to us." If we don't see death or think about it, we can maintain our irrational belief that we are immortal. This avoidance further reinforces our fears.

> I'm amazed how some families say, "Just call me when it's over." They are afraid to watch the death. It's not something you get used to.   Vickie...nurse

If we fear the dying process and stay away, we deny our loved ones and ourselves the experience of being together at one of life's most intimate moments. Theresa Wallace expressed this when she wrote about spending time with her mother during her terminal illness. "Relationships are what give life its deepest meaning and provide the sustenance for us to live fully. Simply being together and enjoying it are the heart and soul of love and life." [1]

Saying Good-bye

Our participation in death is an act of love. It takes courage to stay and say good-bye. When we allow ourselves to be part of the dying process, there is the opportunity to view death as having significance in the natural order of life. If we believe in the resurrection of Jesus Christ, we are able to recognize death as a process that begins from the moment we are born. It is then we can accept death as temporary, knowing we will see our loved ones again.

> I remember my grandmother's death. It happened at home. She had been ill for a very long time. Near the end, friends and relatives came to visit. They sat and held her hand, shared memories, said good-bye. We prepared food for the visitors. In the evening, my mother played the piano, and we all sang hymns to Grandma and cried. It was beautiful.   Leslie...age 56

The sense of belonging that is present when people die at home can be fostered in the nursing-home environment. Facilities have a responsibility, not only to impact the quality of life for residents, but also the quality of their death. They can help the residents let go. They can help the family members say good-bye.

In the past few years, institutions have done a better job of this by providing more support during the dying process. Both private and secular homes now provide pastoral support and hospice care.

> I feel we all try to help the families. Everybody goes out of their way to try to make it a better experience, if they can. We offer counseling, a minister or priest. We can provide them with whatever they need – coffee, food, blankets, someone to talk to.   Chari...nurse

Family members and friends are often uncomfortable with the experience of dying. They may feel embarrassed because they don't know what to say or do. They may be afraid that their grief will be upsetting to the dying person. To be present when death is near, can be difficult, but it can also bring comfort and closure to both family and resident. To sit with a loved one, to hold his hand, to talk to him, even if he can no longer speak or acknowledge your presence, is to show the greatest measure of love. To minister to an individual in this way is to pay tribute to that person's life.

> I spent the last hour of my mother's life reading to her from the beautiful Mother's day cards that she had received a week earlier. She was in a coma. Her eyes were shut. I was crying. Then I noticed a tear running down her cheek, and I knew that she had heard me. Nancy...45

Author Wendy Murray Zoba speaks of being with her father when he died. "To serve my father, to fill his cup with good things as he transferred accounts from this life to the next, this was to me a sacrament. To warm him, to cover his feet, to refresh his dry mouth with lemon-glycerin swabs, to me, was a privilege, and the most profound service one human being can render to another." [2]

Some families want to know the exact moment of death
so that they can come. They forget we can't predict that.
Others come in shifts and take turns staying around the
clock. Sometimes, the resident gets better for a while,
and they have to do it all over again.   Shelly...nurse

In a nursing home, you see it all: people who are afraid
to die, families who can't bear to watch the process and stay
away and the awful isolation of dying alone.

When I know residents are going to die, I try to make
sure they are not alone. I tell them their family loves
them. I tell them that we love them, because we really
do. I talk to them all the time, even after they are gone.
It's just the natural thing to do.   Vickie....nurse

But there is also witness to the beautiful side of life
and death, caregivers who miss their lunch breaks to sit at the
bedside of a dying person.

"A special thank you to the nurse who was with my
mother when she died. I walked in, and she was holding
her hand. That memory will always be in my heart."
Janet...age 47

In the past decade, the subject of life after death has
created much interest. While books on this topic reflect near-
death experiences that are universally common around the
world, they are not unique to life outside the institutional
setting. Caregivers report many instances of unexplainable
happenings.

I remember one truly peaceful death. I had been caring
for a very dignified lady. She was comatose, and we
knew death was imminent. At one point, the woman

opened her eyes and asked me to call a pastor. When he
arrived, she opened her eyes once more but had a far-
away look, as if she could see something that we
couldn't. She would smile, nod her head, and smile
again. Then, she put out her hand and started praying
The Lord's Prayer. She died before she finished.
Nancy...nurse

Many families support their loved ones every day,
from the time they enter the nursing home until they die. This
is truly a gift of love. It enables the family to oversee the care
that is being provided and to maintain the sense of belonging
that we all need so desperately in our lives. As a result,
resident, family and staff become an important part of each
other's lives. When the resident dies, the family and staff
suffer not only the loss of the individual, but also the loss of
their relationship as joint caregivers.

There are families who live far away and have not seen
their loved ones for many years. Some have alienated
themselves because of past conflicts. They may decide to stay
away and not be involved as death nears. Others come at the
end to ease their guilt. The little time they spend is not enough
to reconcile the years of differences, but there can be healing
and forgiveness when they come to say good-bye.

I remember calling a son, who lived far away, to tell
him that his mother was dying. He traveled thousands of
miles across the country to be at her side. Periodically,
he would call us, when he was between planes, to say,
"Tell my mother I'm on my way." We would do this,
and she seemed to understand. When he arrived, the son
sat on her bed and gathered his mother up in his arms
and cradled her. I will never forget the sight of that
grown man, rocking his mother and singing softly to
her, the songs of his childhood.   Sarah...nurse

*And God shall wipe away all tears
from their eyes; and there shall be
no more death, neither sorrow, nor
crying, neither shall there be
anymore pain; for the former things
are passed away.*
(Revelation 21:4)
King James

Suggestions for Families

If you desire to be with your parent or loved one, at the time of death, express your wishes to the nursing staff. Does your family choose to stay around the clock? Do you want younger children to be present? Do you need help in explaining death to them? Ask the staff what provisions are available to make you comfortable. Let them know what you need and how they can help you.

Keep in mind that the dying person often has an acute sense of hearing. Remember to leave the room to discuss sensitive issues. Continue to speak softly to your family member. Read to him, pray with him, or sing his favorite hymns. Hug, kiss, climb in bed with your loved one, if you wish. You won't get another chance.

When the time comes, give your loved one permission to go. Sometimes residents will hold on to life because they sense the grief of their family and don't want to let them down. Say good-bye. Let your parent know that you look forward to the day when you will meet again in eternity.

After death, there is no urgency to remove the body from the facility. Some families choose to stay with their loved one for awhile before letting go. Take your time. This is a perfectly natural way to express grief, and it can bring healing to those involved.

Additional Resources

On Death & Dying, Elizabeth Kubler-Ross, Collier Books 1997.
Helping People Through Grief, Delores Kuenning, Bethany House Publishers, 1987.

Suggested Bible readings:
      1 Corinthians 15: 51-59
      2 Corinthians 5: 1-9
      Thessalonians 4: 13-18,

Endnotes

Chapter 2

1 Barash, David P., *Aging, An Exploration*, University of Washington Press, Seattle and London, 1983, p. 4.

Chapter 3

1 Wylie, Tex Information Aids, *Growing Old In America*, 1994, P. 9.

Chapter 4

1 Wylie, Texas Information Plus, *Profile of The Nation*, 1996, p. 16.

Chapter 5

1 Shield, Renee Rose, *Uneasy Ending, Daily Life In An American Nursing Home*, Cornell University Press, 1988, p. 215.

Chapter 8

1 Littwin, Susan, "A Call For Help, The Untold Story of Elder Abuse Today," *New Choices,* September 1995, p. 36.

2 Ibid.

3 Ibid, p. 37.

Chapter 9

1 Dobihal, Edward F. Jr., and Steward, Charles William, *When A Friend Is Dying*, Abingdon Press, 1984, p. 15.

2 Bayly, Joseph, *The Last Thing We Talk About*, Life Journey Books, 1969, p. 27.

3 Dobihal, Edward F. Jr., and Steward, Charles William, *When A Friend Is Dying*, Abingdon Press, 1984, p. 15.

4 Diamond, Timothy, *Making Grey Gold*, University of Chicago Press, 1992, p. 119.

Chapter 10

1 Wallace, Therese, "To Eleanore," *Runner's World*, November 1994, p. 20.

2 Zoba, Wendy Murray, "How We Die," *Christianity Today*, April 8 1996, p. 34.

Appendix

Alzheimer's Association
Suite 1000
919 North Michigan Avenue
Chicago, IL 60611
(312) 335-8700
Information and referral service: 1-800-272-3900
Web site: http://www.alz.org
This is a voluntary organization that provides support services to families and patients dealing with Alzheimer's disease. They have a toll-free hot line that provides, information to the caller, about local Alzheimer's chapters and resources in the community.

American Association of Retired Persons
601 E Street NW
Washington, DC 20049
(202) 434-2277
Web site: http://www.aarp.org
A non-profit organization dedicated to helping older Americans achieve lives of independence, dignity, and purpose. See their Web site for list of services.

American Hospice Foundation
Suite 700
1130 Connecticut Ave. NW
Washington, DC 20036-4101
(202) 223-0204
Web site: http//www.americanhospice.org

American Parkinson's Disease Association
Suite 4B
1250 Hylan Boulevard
Staten Island, NY 10305
(718) 981-8001
Toll-free Hotline: 1-800-223-2732
This is a volunteer organization that funds research to find a cure for Parkinson's disease, provides public education about the disease, and offers assistance to patients and their families.

Children of Aging Parents
Suite 302-A
1609 Woodbourne Road
Levittown, PA 19057
(215) 945-6900
Toll-Free Information and Referral Service: 1-800-227-7294
This is a non-profit agency that provides information and emotional support to caregivers of older people. Material available for starting a self-help program.

National Association of State Units on Aging
Suite 725
1225 I Street NW
Washington, DC 20005
(202) 898-2578
Eldercare Locator: 1-800-677-1116
Information Service: 1-800-989-6537
A resource for locating your state long-term-care ombudsman program which deals with care issues and residents' rights.

National Citizens' Coalition for Nursing Home Reform
Suite 202
1424 16th Street NW
Washington, DC 20036-2211
(202) 332-2275
The purpose of this organization is to define and achieve quality
for people with long-term-care needs through informed consumers,
effective citizen groups, and ombudsman programs. Support
groups are available in some localities.

Visiting Nurse Associations of America
11 Beacon Street
Suite 910
Boston, MA 02108
Information Service Toll-Free 1-888-866-8773
Supports community-based non-profit home health care providers,
whose purpose is to provide quality care to all people, regardless of
their ability to pay.

ORDER FORM

Code	Title	Price	Qty	Amount
2146PP	In The Care of Strangers	$16.50 ea	_____	$_____
2142PP	Keeping In Touch With the Community ...	$14.50 ea	_____	$_____

State Tax $_____

Shipping, Packing, Handling, Insurance $_____

Total $_____

Order Additional Copies for Friends & Colleagues

By Phone
1/800/551-8783
Office Hours
Monday-Friday,
8:00 am - 5:00 pm

By Mail
Professional Printing & Publishing, Inc.
P.O. Box 5758
Bossier City, LA 71171-5758

By Fax
1/318/746-6995
Our FAX line is open
24 hours a day,
7 days a week

Web Site: http://www.ppandp.com   **E-mail:** order@ppandp.com

SHIP TO:

Name_____

Facility Name _____

Tel. (   ) _____

Street Address_____

City_____State_____ Zip Code _____

☐ Check or Money Order enclosed for total amount.
Make payable to Professional Printing & Publishing, Inc.
Charge My:

☐ Mastercard   ☐ VISA   ☐ Discover   ☐ American Express

Expiration Date: Month_____ Year_____

Signature: _____

(required on all charge orders)

Both authors can be contacted through Dr. Langmade's self-help Web site, Doc
In The Box (http//www.docinthebox.com). Prices effective until 12/31/98.